Emotional Labour in Work with Patients and Clients

Occupational Safety, Health, and Ergonomics: Theory and Practice

Series Editor: Danuta Koradecka
(Central Institute for Labour Protection – National Research Institute)

This series will contain monographs, references, and professional books on a compendium of knowledge in the interdisciplinary area of environmental engineering, which covers ergonomics and safety and the protection of human health in the working environment. Its aim consists in an interdisciplinary, comprehensive and modern approach to hazards, not only those already present in the working environment, but also those related to the expected changes in new technologies and work organizations. The series aims to acquaint both researchers and practitioners with the latest research in occupational safety and ergonomics. The public, who want to improve their own or their family's safety, and the protection of heath will find it helpful, too. Thus, individual books in this series present both a scientific approach to problems and suggest practical solutions; they are offered in response to the actual needs of companies, enterprises, and institutions.

Individual and Occupational Determinants: Work Ability in People with Health Problems
Joanna Bugajska, Teresa Makowiec-Dąbrowska, Tomasz Kostka

Healthy Worker and Healthy Organization: A Resource-Based Approach
Dorota Żołnierczyk-Zreda

Emotional Labour in Work with Patients and Clients: Effects and Recommendations for Recovery
Dorota Żołnierczyk-Zreda

New Opportunities and Challenges in Occupational Safety and Health Management
Daniel Podgórski

Emerging Chemical Risks in the Work Environment
Małgorzata Pośniak

Visual and Non-Visual Effects of Light: Working Environment and Well-Being
Agnieszka Wolska, Dariusz Sawicki, Małgorzata Tafil-Klawe

Occupational Noise and Workplace Acoustics: Advances in Measurement and Assessment Techniques
Dariusz Pleban

Virtual Reality and Virtual Environments: A Tool for Improving Occupational Safety and Health
Andrzej Grabowski

Head, Eye, and Face Personal Protective Equipment: New Trends, Practice and Applications
Katarzyna Majchrzycka

Nanoaerosols, Air Filtering and Respiratory Protection: Science and Practice
Katarzyna Majchrzycka

Microbial Corrosion of Buildings: A Guide to Detection, Health Hazards, and Mitigation
Rafał L. Górny

Respiratory Protection Against Hazardous Biological Agents
Katarzyna Majchrzycka, Justyna Szulc, Małgorzata Okrasa

For more information about this series, please visit: https://www.crcpress.com/
Occupational-Safety-Health-and-Ergonomics-Theory-and-Practice/book-series/CRCOSHETP

Emotional Labour in Work with Patients and Clients

Effects and Recommendations for Recovery

Edited by
Dorota Żołnierczyk-Zreda

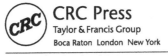

CRC Press
Taylor & Francis Group
Boca Raton London New York

CRC Press is an imprint of the
Taylor & Francis Group, an **informa** business

First edition published 2021
by CRC Press
6000 Broken Sound Parkway NW, Suite 300, Boca Raton, FL 33487-2742

and by CRC Press
2 Park Square, Milton Park, Abingdon, Oxon, OX14 4RN

Library of Congress Cataloging-in-Publication Data

Names: Zolnierczyk-Zreda, Dorota, author.
Title: Emotional labour in work with patients and clients : effects and
recommendations for recovery / Dorota Zolnierczyk-Zreda, Andrzej
Najmiec, Zofia Mockałło, Anna Łukczak, Łukasz Baka.
Description: First edition. | Boca Raton : CRC Press, 2020. | Series:
Occupational safety, health, and ergonomics: theory and practice |
Includes bibliographical references and index.
Identifiers: LCCN 2020007826 (print) | LCCN 2020007827 (ebook) | ISBN
9780367900953 (hbk) | ISBN 9780367513719 (paperback) | ISBN
9781003032496 (ebk)
Subjects: LCSH: Job stress. | Burnout (Psychology) | Medical personnel--Job
stress. | Human services personnel--Job stress.
Classification: LCC HF5548.85 .Z65 2020 (print) | LCC HF5548.85 (ebook) |
DDC 158.7/2--dc23
LC record available at https://lccn.loc.gov/2020007826
LC ebook record available at https://lccn.loc.gov/2020007827

ISBN: 9780367900953 (hbk)
ISBN: 9781003032496 (ebk)

Typeset in Times
by Deanta Global Publishing Services, Chennai, India

Contents

Acknowledgment

Wishing a special thank you to Paulina Barańska for translating this book into English.

Series Editor

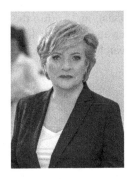

Professor Danuta Koradecka, PhD, DMed and Director of the Central Institute for Labour Protection – National Research Institute (CIOP-PIB), is a specialist in occupational health. Her research interests include the human health effects of hand-transmitted vibration; ergonomics research on the human body's response to the combined effects of vibration, noise, low temperature and static load; assessment of static and dynamic physical load; development of hygienic standards as well as development and implementation of ergonomic solutions to improve working conditions in accordance with International Labour Organisation (ILO) convention and European Union (EU) directives. She is the author of over 200 scientific publications and several books on occupational safety and health.

***

The "Occupational Safety, Health, and Ergonomics: Theory and Practice" series of monographs is focused on the challenges of the 21st century in this area of knowledge. These challenges address diverse risks in the working environment of chemical (including carcinogens, mutagens, endocrine agents), biological (bacteria, viruses), physical (noise, electromagnetic radiation) and psychophysical (stress) nature. Humans have been in contact with all these risks for thousands of years. Initially, their intensity was lower, but over time it has gradually increased, and now too often exceeds the limits of man's ability to adapt. Moreover, risks to human safety and health, so far assigned to the working environment, are now also increasingly emerging in the living environment. With the globalisation of production and merging of labour markets, the practical use of the knowledge on occupational safety, health, and ergonomics should be comparable between countries. The presented series will contribute to this process.

The Central Institute for Labour Protection – National Research Institute, conducting research in the discipline of environmental engineering, in the area of working environment and implementing its results, has summarised the achievements – including its own – in this field from 2011 to 2019. Such work would not be possible without cooperation with scientists from other Polish and foreign institutions as authors or reviewers of this series. I would like to express my gratitude to all of them for their work.

It would not be feasible to publish this series without the professionalism of the specialists from the Publishing Division, the Centre for Scientific Information and Documentation, and the International Cooperation Division of our Institute. The challenge was also the editorial compilation of the series and ensuring the efficiency of this publishing process, for which I would like to thank the entire editorial team of CRC Press–Taylor & Francis.

***

This monograph, published in 2020, has been based on the results of a research task carried out within the scope of the second to fourth stage of the Polish National Programme "Improvement of safety and working conditions" partly supported — within the scope of research and development — by the Ministry of Science and Higher Education/National Centre for Research and Development, and within the scope of state services — by the Ministry of Family, Labour and Social Policy. The Central Institute for Labour Protection – National Research Institute is the Programme's main coordinator and contractor.

Editor

Dorota Żołnierczyk-Zreda, PhD, Head of Laboratory of Social Psychology, Central Institute for Labour Protection – National Research Institute, Warsaw, Poland, is a senior researcher in occupational health psychology. Her research is focused on psychosocial working conditions and mental health at work, its determinants and various methods to sustain it in different groups of workers (e.g. young, older) and different occupational groups. She has extensive experience in qualitative studies and quantitative studies as well as in policy research and monitoring studies. She is also involved in national and international projects investigating different stress management interventions on both the organizational and individual levels. She is the author or co-author of approximately 60 scientific publications, including articles, chapters in monographs and textbooks, and many speeches at scientific conferences nationally and abroad. She is a licensed cognitive-behavioral therapist.

Contributors

Łukasz Baka, PhD, DSc, is a senior researcher in occupational health psychology at the Laboratory of Social Psychology, Central Institute for Labour Protection – National Research Institute, Warsaw, Poland; member of PEROSH Prolonging Working Life Initiative. His research focuses on psychosocial work conditions and its consequences on mental health and organizational behavior. He is the author or co-author of seven books and over 50 scientific articles related to the subjects.

Anna Łuczak, PhD, is an occupational psychologist at the Laboratory of Social Psychology, Central Institute for Labour Protection – National Research Institute, Warsaw, Poland, who specializes in transport psychology. Her research is focused on stress and mental load at work, difficult and dangerous jobs, job selection including psychological drivers' testing and adaptation of the psychological tests used in job selection to Polish conditions, and assessment of work capacity of people with disabilities.

Zofia Mockałło, MA, is a researcher at the Laboratory of Social Psychology, Central Institute for Labour Protection – National Research Institute, Warsaw, Poland, and a member of PEROSH Wellbeing at Work Initiative. Her research area is focused on work and organizational psychology, and sources and effects of employees' wellbeing, with special interest in psychosocial job demands and resources.

Andrzej Najmiec, MA, is a researcher at the Laboratory of Social Psychology, Central Institute for Labour Protection – National Research Institute, Warsaw, Poland. His research area is focused on psychosocial working conditions with special interest in stress and social support, work and organizational psychology, transport psychology, and safety culture.

1 Emotional Labor at Work with Patients and Customers

The Effects and Recommendations for Recovery

Dorota Żołnierczyk-Zreda

The tertiary sector, or services sector, has become the largest sector of the economy in the Western world, and is also the fastest-growing sector. The services economy currently contributes to approximately 70% of the gross domestic product (GDP) in the US and in European countries [The World Factbook 2017]. The work of a significant number of persons employed in this sector often requires intensive contact with customers or patients, where emotional labor is a job demand. It means that workers have to display certain emotions at work, while suppressing other feelings, according to the emotional display rules set by the employer [Hochschild 1983; Côté 2005]. Therefore, emotional labor encompasses a process that includes (a) explicit emotional demands (i.e. display rules) and (b) the effortful strategies needed to meet those demands (i.e. emotion regulation) [Diefendorff and Gosserand 2003; Grandey and Sayre 2019].

The research presented in this monograph covers two service sector branches: health care/social services and public administration, both of which are characterized by high emotional labor demands, and where display rules are explicitly communicated to motivate an effective interpersonal performance [Diefendorff, Richard, and Croyle 2006; Grandey and Sayre 2019]. The health care sector includes 'social mission' occupations that are based on the provision of physical and health security, satisfying the basic needs of other people, as well as providing basic skills or knowledge, enabling patients to function in society. The main motivation of workers employed in this sector should therefore be the willingness to help and care for others. The other sector employs tax, revenue, and private or social insurance workers. The main objective of the work performed in this sector is to satisfy the needs of customers by providing high-quality customer service and/or to persuade the customer to purchase the most profitable product from the organization's point of view, i.e. "service with a smile" [Chua, Bakerb, and Murmann 2012].

1

An important part of the work of persons employed in both sectors is emotional regulation aimed at expression of certain emotions (e.g. sympathy, compassion, enthusiasm) or suppression of feelings (e.g. irritation, anger, hostility). However, interpersonal interactions with patients and customers induce a variety of both positive and negative emotions in workers [Dormann and Zapf 2004; Grandey, Diefendorff, and Rupp 2012; Grandey and Sayre 2019]. Being compassionate may be difficult when the patient (sometimes involuntarily) is offensive or even aggressive, or when a customer is overdemanding. Thus, there will be instances when workers experience emotions different in type or intensity from that prescribed by the emotional display rules. This discrepancy between the actual feeling and that required by the emotional display rules has been named 'emotional dissonance' by Holman, Iñigo, and Totterdell [2008]. Hochschild [1983] revealed that when the emotions and feelings of workers do not match the emotional display rules and the workers experience 'emotional dissonance', they often use one of two emotional regulation strategies to ensure that their actions are in line with the required emotional conduct. The first strategy is deep acting, which alters the emotion felt in order to change it and produce a genuine emotional display; the other is surface acting, which only modifies the outward expression of the emotion and produces a faked emotional display. According to Grandey and Sayre [2019], deep acting refers to modifying feelings, which can be done using cognitive strategies (e.g. refocusing attention, reappraisal) to proactively change how one feels (e.g. taking a difficult client's perspective to genuinely show concern). Surface acting is a type of behavioral modulation (e.g. suppression, amplifying), often performed reactively to negative events (e.g. hiding irritation with a difficult customer).

Deep acting has been found to have a positive association with personal accomplishment and job satisfaction [Bono and Vey 2005; Hülsheger and Schewe 2011], whereas surface acting, accompanied by the lack of authenticity, or expressing emotions differently or in opposition to those actually felt, may constitute a source of stress, because it involves internal tension and suppression of feelings [Brotheridge and Grandey 2002]. It is believed that surface acting requires more effort than deep acting [Richards and Gross 2000] and may with time lead to a disconnection from one's true emotions and instead to feelings of others, and to emotional exhaustion, as well as reduced self-esteem [Brotheridge and Grandey 2002]. To explain this mechanism, particularly the negative effects of emotional labor, the demands and resources theory, such as the Conservation of Resources Theory [Hobfoll 1998; Brotheridge and Lee 2002] or demand–resource model of job burnout [Demerouti et al. 2001] are frequently used. According to these theories, an effort demanding surface acting results in depletion of personal resources, both physical and psychological. However, it has been suggested that, while surface acting may directly deplete effort, deep acting may positively affect well-being due to its role in promoting and obtaining resources [Holman, Iñigo, and Totterdell 2008]. Self-authenticity has been found to be a significant mechanism of the effects of deep acting on worker well-being [Brotheridge and Lee 2002].

Despite the significant knowledge of the different effects of emotional labor, much remains to be explored. The purpose of this monograph is to fill some of these gaps in the contemporary research. The research presented in the monograph demonstrates, for example, that levels of deep and surface acting vary considerably between occupations and contexts, and that contextual factors (such as hostile customer behaviors, or organization type: public or private) appear to play a significant role in the adoption of deep and surface strategies and their effects on worker well-being. The studies presented in the monograph reveal also certain individual factors, such as self-efficacy, that can mitigate the negative effects of emotional labor.

Much has been established on the impact of emotional labor on psychological well-being, such as job burnout and job satisfaction, however, there is still little data on these effects at the level of physical health or lifestyle. This monograph presents research that shows that long-term exposure to high emotional demands at work can lead to depression, and that it can result in excessive alcohol consumption and physical inactivity, which can also reduce the resilience to stress associated with caring for patients.

The monograph also covers methods that can increase this resilience and mitigate the negative effects of emotional labor, including solutions at the level of organizations, in which employees have intensive contacts with patients and customers.

In a study conducted by Mockałło carried out among public tax administration workers and described in Chapter 2, "Stress-Inducing Customer Behaviors and Wellbeing in Tax Administration Workers: What Is the Role of Emotional Labor?", the author has investigated whether these persons, when confronted with stress-inducing customer behaviors (disproportionate customer expectations and hostile customer behaviors), would choose the deep or surface acting strategy (two aspects of surface acting were examined: hiding feelings and faking emotions). The study has also examined whether deep acting would result in a lower level of job burnout (disengagement from work and exhaustion) and improved physical health, examining symptoms such as headaches, nausea, weakness, stomach problems, etc. The study results have proven that the more workers are confronted with stress-inducing customer behaviors, the more exhausted they feel, the less engaged they are, and the poorer their physical health is. This data is yet further evidence of the negative relationship between stress-inducing customer behaviors and job burnout, and physical symptoms, the latter less frequently analyzed in the literature. Moreover, the study has revealed that deep acting is not associated with job burnout, but significant relationships have been observed with regard to physical health. The result may suggest that persons who perform deep acting emotional labor enjoy job satisfaction and personal accomplishment; however, handling difficult customers with the deep acting strategy continues to drain these workers of personal resources and energy. Contrary to the hypothesis, in conditions of stress-inducing customer behaviors, tax administration workers used both deep and surface acting strategies. Nevertheless, the effort of deep acting led to physical symptoms felt by these workers, which had not been reported in the literature so far. A further novelty of this research is a distinction between two surface acting aspects that are associated with physical symptoms in different ways. In terms of worker mental and physical well-being, hiding feelings has proven to be a weaker type of emotional regulation: it has been found to be associated with poorer physical and psychological health (burnout), while faking emotions has been positively related to job burnout only. In general, the results of this study indicate that even in emotionally difficult situations, workers apply all forms of emotional labor, and that the effects of this labor have various impacts on the mental and physical well-being of workers.

Interesting results with respect to the effects of deep and surface acting on physical and mental health, as well as on job burnout, have also been revealed in the Najmiec's study carried out among private and public insurance workers who were confronted with excessive demands and hostile customer behaviors as presented in Chapter 3: "The Relationship between Intensification of Stress-Inducing Customer Behaviors, Job Burnout, and Well-Being of Customer Service Workers: The Role of Emotional Labor Types". Namely, it has been found that among private insurance workers, in conditions of frequent exposure to hostile customer behaviors, the worst physical and mental well-being was experienced by those employees who performed the highest levels of deep acting, compared to those who used the surface acting strategy. Different results were obtained in the group of social insurance workers. In conditions of high-intensity hostile customer behaviors, those employees who performed deep acting emotional labor in customer interactions were characterized by a better physical and mental well-being than those using surface acting. Also, in conditions of disproportionate customer expectations, the greatest physical and mental well-being, as well as the lowest level of exhaustion, were observed among employees using the deep acting strategy. The overall effect of deep acting on job burnout was negative: the more often deep acting was used, the lower the level of job burnout was observed in the group of both private and public insurance workers.

Baka has conducted a cross-lagged study among workers of social rehabilitation centers – youth education centers, youth sociotherapy centers, youth hostels, and correctional facilities – which is described in Chapter 4: "Health Impairment Process in Human Service Work: The Role of Emotional Demands and Personal Resources". The researcher has examined whether emotional and hiding emotions demands are associated with depression, and the role job burnout and self-efficacy play in this relationship. It has been found that job demands are directly related to depression measured after a year since the first measurement. However, a mediation effects analysis has shown that job burnout plays a key role in the development of depression. High job demands lead to an increase in the job burnout measured after a year, which also exacerbates depression. The author concludes that emotional demands occurring in the work environment affect the workers in a long-term manner, and their effects are postponed [Hockey 1997]. In the first phase of coping with these demands, the worker mobilizes the strength, commitment, and effort needed to perform professional tasks in order to maintain the required level of work quality. This gradually exhausts the worker's resources to cope with stress, resulting in job burnout and then mental problems, such as depression. The beneficial function of personal resources, i.e. self-efficacy, has also been partially confirmed. A high self-efficacy mediated the negative effect of hiding emotions demands (but not emotional demands) on job burnout. The obtained study results, alongside the scientific value, carry important knowledge that can be used in psychological practice. The results reveal that strengthening the self-efficacy of employees facing high emotional demands in their work should be a necessary component of programs preventing job burnout and possible depression.

Najmiec has conducted a study among 200 employees of residential care establishments whose work is based on intensive and direct contact with the sick, elderly, and persons with chronic mental illnesses or intellectual disabilities, as presented in Chapter 5: "Determinants and Consequences of Work-Related Stress in Personnel of Residential Care Establishments". The majority of the surveyed workers (over 70%) believed that their work always required addressing the problems of others, putting the workers in emotionally difficult situations. One third reported that their work did not give them the opportunity to develop their skills and learn new competences. They experienced unwanted conduct from patients, such as threats of physical violence or even violence itself, irritating behavior and unwelcome sexual interest. Most of the surveyed workers also reported musculoskeletal disorders resulting from the frequent lifting of chronically ill patients. Among the activities aimed at coping with such job demands, the author has mentioned relaxation training, aggression handling training, and reduction of contradictory job demands such as the need for empathy toward the sick while "not taking up" their complaints.

In Łuczak's study carried out among medical staff of psychiatric and addiction treatment wards and described in Chapter 6:"Psychosocial Stressors at Work and Stress Prevention Methods among Medical Staff of Psychiatric and Addiction Treatment Wards", the most important stressors have been found to be high emotional demands and patient aggression. At the lifestyle level, the surveyed workers also reported a lack of physical activity during leisure time as well as alcohol abuse, which could be a result of the stress induced by high emotional job demands, but which also potentially reduces the employees' ability to cope with this stress. The author recommends that support programs addressed to this occupational group should include such methods of proven effectiveness as Mindfulness-Based Stress Reduction (MBSR) training, Promoting Adult Resilience (PAR) training, emotional intelligence training, the education of all psychiatric ward staff members on escalated aggression processes, the anticipation of violence and effective intervention at various stages of aggression, as well as programs aimed at alcohol abuse prevention among the medical personnel of psychiatric and addiction treatment wards.

Generally, the research presented in this monograph shows how the effects of emotional labor can differ between employees, but above all that there are many methods to deal with these effects and, even better, to counteract them before they appear.

REFERENCES

Bono, J. E., and M. A. Vey. 2005. Toward understanding emotional management at work: A quantitative review of emotional labor research. In *Emotions in Organizational Behavior*, eds. C. E. J. Härtel, W. J. Zerbe, and N. M. Ashkanasy, 213–233. Mahwah, NJ: Lawrence Erlbaum.

Brotheridge, C. M., and A. A. Grandey. 2002. Emotional labor and burnout: Comparing two perspectives of "people work". *J Vocat Behav* 60:17–39.

Brotheridge, C. M., and R. T. Lee. 2002. Testing a conservation of resources model of the dynamics of emotional labor. *J Occup Health Psychol* 7:57–67.

Chua, K. H., M. A. Bakerb, and S. K. Murrmann. 2012. When we are onstage, we smile: The effects of emotional labor on employee work outcomes. *Int J Hosp Manag* 31:906–915.

Côté, S. 2005. A social interaction model of the effects of emotion regulation on work strain. *Acad Manag Rev* 30:509–530.

Demerouti, E., A. B. Bakker, F. Nachreiner, and W. B. Schaufeli. 2001. The job demands–resources model of burnout. *J Appl Psychol* 86:499–512.

Diefendorff, J. M., and R. H. Gosserand. 2003. Understanding the emotional labour process: A control theory perspective. *J Organ Behav* 24:945–59.

Diefendorff, J. M., E. M. Richard, and M. H. Croyle. 2006. Are emotional display rules formal job requirements? Examination of employee and supervisor perceptions. *J Occup Organ Psychol* 79):273–298.

Dormann, C., and D. Zapf. 2004. Customer-related social stressors and burnout. *J Occup Health Psychol* 9:61–82.

Grandey, A. A., J. M. Diefendorff, and D. E. Rupp. 2012. *Emotional Labor in the 21st Century: Diverse Perspectives on Emotion Regulation at Work*. New York: Routledge.

Grandey, A., and G. M. Sayre. 2019. Emotional labor: Regulating emotions for a wage. *Curr Dir Psychol Sci* 28(2):096372141881277.

Hobfoll, S. E. 1998. *Stress, Culture and Community: The Psychology and Philosophy of Stress*. New York: Plenum.

Hochschild, A. R. 1983. *The Managed Heart: Commercialization of Human Feeling*. Berkeley, CA: University of California Press.

Hockey, G. J. 1997. Compensatory control in the regulation of human performance under stress and high workload: A cognitive-energetical framework. *Biol Psychol* 45:73–93.

Holman, D., D. Martinez-Iñigo, and P. Totterdell. 2008. Emotional labor and employee well-being: An integrative review. In *Research Companion to Emotion in Organizations*, eds. N. M. Ashkanasy, and C. L. Cooper, 301–315. Cheltenham, UK: Edward Elgar.

Hülsheger, U. R., and A. F. Schewe. 2011. On the costs and benefits of emotional labor: A meta-analysis of three decades of research. *J Occup Health Psychol* 16:361–389.

Richards, J. M., and J. J. Gross. 2000. Emotional regulation and memory: The cognitive costs of keeping one's cool. *J Pers Soc Psychol* 79:410–24.

The World Factbook – Central Intelligence Agency. 2017. Central Intelligence Agency. www.cia.gov/library/publications/the-world-factbook (accessed 20September 2017).

2 Stress-Inducing Customer Behaviors and Wellbeing in Tax Administration Workers

What Is the Role of Emotional Labor?

Zofia Mockałło

CONTENTS

2.1 INTRODUCTION

Customer service work involves specific psychosocial risks and has been of interest to researchers for many years. A particular psychosocial risk factor in this occupational group is the direct customer contact, entailing various emotional demands. According to the latest EWCS report, in the European Union, 31% of workers are expected to hide feelings at work at all times, or nearly at all times [Parent-Thirion et al. 2017]. The highest percentage of employees who are confronted with such job demands work in the services sector: health care (44%), public administration (38%), education (36%), retail and hospitality (36%), and finance (35%). In these sectors, workers also face customer anger more frequently than the EU average. At least three quarters of the working time is spent on handling abusive customers in the following sectors: healthcare (26%), education (22%), retail and hospitality (20%), finance (19%), and public administration (17%) [Parent-Thirion et al. 2017]. Lastly, emotionally demanding conditions make up three quarters of the working time for 22% of healthcare workers, 13% of public administration workers, and 11% of education workers.

According to the Statistics Poland (GUS) data [GUS 2014], the highest number of workers exposed to violence or threats of violence, and bullying or intimidation at the workplace (one or both factors) was recorded in the "public administration and national defense" and "social and health insurance" sectors (7.4% of workers), followed by the "administration and social services" sector (6.9% of workers). Such a high workplace bullying rate suggests that these sectors' workers are much more exposed to stressful interactions with customers, or high emotional demands at work.

2.1.1 STRESS-INDUCING CUSTOMER BEHAVIORS AND WORKER WELLBEING

Customer contacts can be a significant source of negative emotions experienced by workers, intensifying work-related stress and potentially leading to job burnout [Kern and Grandey 2009; Dormann and Zapf 2004]. A study by Singh, Goolsby and Rhoads [1994] showed that the level of job burnout in the customer service employee group was higher than in other groups usually associated with job burnout, such as police officers and nurses. In a study conducted in different groups of customer service workers, the most stress-inducing customer behaviors were disproportionate expectations, customer aversion, verbal aggression and ambiguous expectations [Dormann and Zapf 2004]. Difficult interactions with customers lead to negative emotions [Bazińska and Szczygieł, 2012]. Previous research has proved that interpersonal mistreatment from customers was the most frequent cause of anger and emotional tension among workers [Grandey, Tam, and Brauburger 2002].

Referring to the *Conservation of Resource Theory* [COR, Hobfoll 1989], hostile customer behaviors can be viewed as social stressors that deplete the emotional and cognitive resources of workers, which has a negative impact on their wellbeing [Kern and Grandey 2009]. It has been proved that aggressive customer behavior may be associated with job burnout, the emotional exhaustion of workers, lower-quality customer service, mishandling of customers, poorer performance, absenteeism, tardiness, stress, poor job satisfaction, and intention to quit the job [van Jaarsveld et al. 2010; Sliter, Sliter, and Jex 2012; Adams and Webster 2013; Wilson and Holmvall 2013; Hur, Moon, and Jung 2015; in: Han, Bonn, and Cho 2016].

Zapf et al. (2003) drew attention to the phenomenon of emotional dissonance in the call center industry, where workers had to express positive emotions toward customers, despite experiencing a divergent emotional status. This phenomenon, present not only in the call center industry but in all professions related to customer service work, has been linked to emotional labor [Hochschild 1983].

2.1.2 EMOTIONAL LABOR

One approach to emotional labor is *employee-focused emotional labor*, defined in terms of emotion management and expression aimed at meeting the job demands. This approach measures the emotional dissonance that occurs when the worker expresses feelings other than those actually felt, and the emotion-regulatory processes, such as modifying the expressed emotion, to fulfill the job demands [Brotheridge 2002b]. There have been identified two forms of employee-oriented emotional labor: surface acting and deep acting [Hochschild 1983].

2.1.2.1 Surface Acting

Surface acting emotional labor involves an self-control of expressed emotions e.g. when an employee is smiling despite a bad mood or handling a cumbersome customer. The emotion has been altered, however, the modification takes place uniquely at the behavioral level. Such a faked expression of emotions, different or opposite to those actually felt, constitutes a significant source of stress, because it is associated with internal tension and suppression of genuine feelings. Faking emotions can lead in the long run to a disconnection from one's true emotions and the feelings of others, emotional exhaustion, and reduced self-esteem [Brotheridge 2002b].

2.1.2.2 Deep Acting

Deep acting emotional labor is a process of controlling and modifying emotions to fulfill the officially set emotional display requirements at work [Hochschild 1983]. The emotional regulation is aimed at reducing the perceived dissonance and can lead to a sense of achievement when the goal is reached (e.g. customer satisfaction). Deep acting may not lead to emotional exhaustion as it aims to reduce tension and internal dissonance [Szczygieł et al. 2009]. On the contrary, deep acting emotional labor may be conducive to a lower depersonalization level and a greater sense of accomplishment [Brotheridge 2002b]. Examples of such emotional regulation include a shift in the cognitive perspective (taking the other person's point of view) or a positive refocus, i.e. focusing attention on positive aspects to regulate emotions [Gross 1998; in: Grandey, Dickter, and Sin 2004].

Emotional labor is a job demand particularly characteristic of customer service professions that involve a high intensity of customer contact, the need to maintain visual and/or verbal contact in communication with customers, the expectation to express certain emotions toward customers (e.g. joy), and the presence of official emotional conduct rules (e.g. rules forbidding to show impatience with a customer) [Hochschild 1983].

2.1.3 THE EFFECTS OF EMOTIONAL LABOR

Previous research has shown that emotional labor, particularly surface acting, can be a source of stress, reduced job satisfaction, emotional exhaustion or job burnout [Szczygieł et al. 2009; Brotheridge 2002b; Zammuner and Galli 2005; Kong and Jeon 2018; Rathi, Bhatnagar, and Mishra 2013]. This has been attributed to the substantial effort invested in regulating emotions, which may deplete personal resources [Hochschild 1983]. However, the consequences of emotional labor can also be positive. For example, deep acting has been associated with a sense of personal accomplishment [Brotheridge and Lee 2003; in: Szczygieł et al. 2009], explained by an increased worker perception of self-efficacy, whereby employees begin to identify their behavior as conforming to the standards set by the employer.

The positive consequences of emotional labor are particularly visible at organizational level: emotional labor increases worker performance and customer satisfaction [Szczygieł et al. 2009]. Nonetheless, such an outcome has also been mainly associated with deep acting emotional labor, which seems to be crucial, because customers can detect faked emotions resulting from surface acting emotional labor [Grandey et al. 2005; in: Szczygieł et al. 2009]. A study conducted in a group of female and male nurses has revealed that deep and surface acting differ in terms of the effects on job satisfaction and worker–customer orientation. Deep acting was found to be unrelated to job satisfaction; however, it was associated with a lesser customer (patient) orientation. In turn, surface acting was associated with poorer job satisfaction; however, it correlated with a greater patient orientation [Gountas et al. 2014]. Deep acting emotional labor was also conducive to improved communication between patients and medical personnel, whereas faked emotions were negatively associated with mutual understanding and joint decision-making [Lee, Lovell, and Brotheridge 2010].

2.1.4 PRESENT STUDY

Previous research has shown that deep acting emotional labor is generally 'healthier' for customer service workers: it leads to a sense of accomplishment or protects against depersonalization, while surface acting leads to job burnout. However, when faced with stress-inducing customer behaviors, will deep acting emotional labor also guarantee a better functioning of workers? Will a worker exposed to a stress-inducing customer behavior choose surface or deep acting strategy? The aim of the present research has been to investigate the relationship between stress-inducing customer behaviors, emotional labor and job burnout, and the physical wellbeing of workers. The study has been conducted in a group of tax administration workers, characterized by high exposure to emotional labor job demands, hostile customer behaviors, and hiding feelings' demands. Also, this employee group has not been of interest to researchers so far.

2.1.4.1 Hypotheses

1. Stress-inducing customer behaviors are positively associated with job burnout, and negatively associated with the physical wellbeing of workers.
2. Stress-inducing customer behaviors are positively associated with surface acting, and negatively associated with deep acting emotional labor.
3. Emotional labor is a mediator in the relationship between stress-inducing customer behaviors and the job burnout of workers:
   3a. Deep acting is a mediator in the relationship between stress-inducing customer behaviors (disproportionate customer expectations and hostile behaviors) and job burnout (disengagement from work and exhaustion) of workers: stress-inducing customer behaviors are related negatively to deep acting, which, in turn, is positively associated with job burnout among workers;
   3b. Surface acting (hiding feelings and faking emotions) is a mediator in the relationship between stress-inducing customer behaviors (disproportionate customer expectations and hostile behaviors) and job burnout of workers (disengagement from work and exhaustion): stress-inducing customer behaviors are positively related to surface acting, which, in turn, is positively related to job burnout among workers.
4. Emotional labor is a mediator in the relationship between stress-inducing customer behaviors and the physical wellbeing of workers:
   4a. Deep acting is a mediator in the relationship between stress-inducing customer behaviors (disproportionate customer expectations and hostile behaviors) and the physical wellbeing of workers: stress-inducing customer behaviors are negatively associated with deep acting, which, in turn, is negatively associated with the physical wellbeing of workers;
   4b. Surface acting (hiding feelings and faking emotions) is a mediator in the relationship between stress-inducing customer behaviors (disproportionate customer expectations and hostile behaviors) and the physical wellbeing of workers: stress-inducing customer behaviors are positively associated with surface acting, which, in turn, is negatively associated with the physical wellbeing of workers.

2.2 METHOD

2.2.1 PARTICIPANTS AND PROCEDURE

The study included 403 tax administration workers. These were employees who occupied lower, non-management positions in the organizational hierarchy, and had constant, daily contact with customers. The average daily working time with customers in the study group was 6.21 hours.

The mean age in the study group was 41.7 years ($SD = 9.07$; $Min = 19$; $Max = 68$). Women made up most of the group (351 persons). 65.5% of respondents had a higher education degree, 20.8% had completed post-secondary or incomplete higher education, and 20% had completed secondary vocational education. The average professional career length was 9.63 years ($SD = 7.62$; $Min = 1$; $Max = 55$). The most common type of employment contract in the study group was a permanent work contract – this type of contract was declared by 73% of the group. 12.9% of the group worked on a fixed-term contract basis, and 11.2% were contractors.

The cross-sectional questionnaire survey was carried out, whereby the respondents filled out the questionnaires using the Paper and Pencil Interview (PAPI) technique. The questionnaires were filled out anonymously and after their completion study participants handed over the questionnaires in closed envelopes to the interviewers.

2.2.2 MEASURES

1. *The Stress-Inducing Customer Behavior Scale* (SSZK) [Szczygieł and Bazińska 2013] was used to measure the severity of stress-inducing customer behaviors occurring in interactions with customer service workers. It comprises 12 statements and contains 2 subscales:
   - Hostile customer behaviors (hostile attitudes and negative emotions displayed by customers when interacting with workers),
   - Disproportionate customer expectations (difficult to meet, unclear or excessive, i.e. exceeding standard service or customer expectations).
   The reliability of the tool has been high: the Cronbach's $\alpha = 0.80$ for each subscale.
2. The *Deep Acting and Surface Acting Scale* (SPGPE) [Finogenow, Wróbel, and Mróz 2015] was used to measure emotional labor – deep acting emotional labor and two aspects of surface acting (hiding feelings and faking emotions). The scale comprises nine questions, which are answered on a five-point scale (from "never" to "always"). The Cronbach's α for each subscale has been: 0.67 (deep acting subscale), 0.80 (the hiding-feelings subscale) and 0.72 (the faking-emotions subscale).
3. *The Oldenburg Burnout Inventory Questionnaire* (OLBI) [Demerouti et al. 2003] was used to measure job burnout. The questionnaire comprises 16 statements and contains 2 job burnout scales: exhaustion and disengagement from work. The answer format is a four-point answer scale, where '1' means 'I agree' and '4' means 'I do not agree'. Previous analyses have

shown that both exhaustion and disengagement from work scales are characterized by a satisfactory reliability, Cronbach's $\alpha = 0.73$ and 0.69, respectively [Baka 2015].

4. *The Psychosocial Working Conditions Questionnaire* (Kwestionariusz Psychospołeczne Warunki Pracy, PWP) [Cieślak and Widerszal-Bazyl 2000] was used to measure physical wellbeing, defined as a general assessment of physical health, and the incidence of somatic complaints (headaches, nausea, weakness, stomach problems, etc.).

2.2.3 STATISTICAL ANALYSIS

In order to examine the mediating role of the emotional labor in the relationship between stress-inducing customer behavior and worker wellbeing, a series of mediation analysis with three mediators (*deep acting, faking emotions, hiding feelings*) was conducted using the SPSS 23 Macro Process with bootstrapping (5,000 bootstrap samples; Model 4) [Hayes 2017].

2.3 RESULTS

The correlation analysis (Table 2.1) has shown that both disproportionate customer expectation and hostile customer behaviors are associated with job burnout (disengagement from work and exhaustion) and physical wellbeing: the greater the experience of hostile customer behaviors, the higher the level of job burnout symptoms, and the poorer the physical wellbeing of workers. Age has been significantly associated with hiding feelings: the older the respondent's age, the more frequent their hiding of feelings, as well as the higher their exhaustion, and the poorer their physical wellbeing.

2.3.1 THE MEDIATING ROLE OF EMOTIONAL LABOR IN THE RELATIONSHIP BETWEEN STRESS-INDUCING CUSTOMER BEHAVIORS AND JOB BURNOUT OF WORKERS

2.3.1.1 Disproportionate Customer Expectations and Employee Disengagement from Work

The tested model fit the data ($F(4.398) = 8.16$; $p < 0.001$) and explained 8% of the dependent variable variance. Disproportionate customer expectations were positively associated with disengagement from work: the more the workers were confronted with disproportionate customer expectations, the higher the level of employee disengagement from work was observed, confirming hypothesis 1.

The relationship between the independent variable and the dependent variable remained significant after introducing the mediators into the model; however, it was slightly weakened (Figure 2.1). Disproportionate customer expectations were positively associated with all the analyzed types of emotional labor, which only partially confirmed hypothesis 2.

TABLE 2.1

Descriptive Statistics and Correlations of the Study Variables (N = 403)

	M	SD	Min	Max	1	2	3	4	5	6	7	8	9
1. Age	41.69	9.07	19.00	68.00	—								
2. Hostile behaviors	19.33	5.39	6.00	30.00	0.08	—							
3. Disproportionate customer expectations	21.65	4.44	6.00	30.00	0.05	0.75***	—						
4. Deep acting	2.71	0.78	1.00	4.33	0.05	0.14**	0.15**	—					
5. Hiding feelings	2.87	0.89	1.00	5.00	0.17***	0.11*	0.22***	0.28***	—				
6. Faking emotions	2.39	0.79	1.00	4.67	0.08	0.25***	0.17***	0.36***	0.55***	—			
7. Disengagement from work	2.43	0.45	1.13	3.88	0.05	0.30***	0.28***	-0.06	0.15**	0.30***	—		
8. Exhaustion	2.45	0.51	1.00	3.88	0.18***	0.32***	0.27***	0.08	0.21***	0.29***	0.72***	—	
9. Physical wellbeing	3.68	0.59	1.55	4.91	-0.19***	-0.19***	-0.8***	-0.18***	-0.20***	-0.12*	-0.29***	-0.52***	—

$*** p < 0.001. ** p < 0.01. * p < 0.05.$

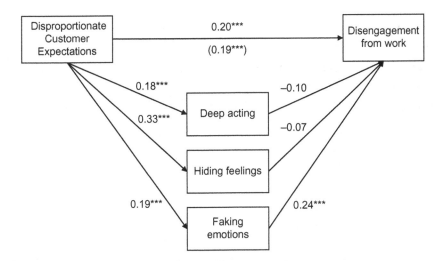

FIGURE 2.1 Regression coefficients of the relationship between disproportionate customer expectations and disengagement from work, mediated by emotional labor. ***$p < 0.001$. **$p < 0.01$. *$p < 0.05$.

The indirect effects analysis (Table 2.2) has shown that the faking emotions factor is a partial mediator in the relationship between disproportionate customer expectations and disengagement from work: disproportionate customer expectations are associated with a more frequent faking of emotions, which leads to a greater disengagement from work. This result has partially supported the hypothesis 3b, however, has not supported the hypothesis 3a.

2.3.1.2 Disproportionate Customer Expectations and Worker Exhaustion

The tested model had a good data fit ($F(4.398) = 20.003$; $p < 0.001$) and explained 17% of the dependent variable variance. Disproportionate customer expectations have been positively associated with worker exhaustion, which has confirmed hypothesis 1 (Figure 2.2).

The relationship between the independent variable and the dependent variable remained significant and was even reinforced, after the introduction of the mediators into the model, which suggests the occurrence of a mechanism of suppression. The indirect effects analysis (Table 2.3) showed that the two aspects of surface acting – hiding feelings and faking emotions – partially explained those dependencies. Disproportionate customer expectations have been associated with greater exhaustion, which has been partly explained by the use of the surface-acting strategy. These results have partially supported hypothesis 3b – except that instead of the assumed mediation mechanism, a mechanism of suppression has been observed – but have not supported hypothesis 3a.

2.3.1.3 Hostile Customer Behaviors and Employee Disengagement from Work

The tested model fit the data ($F(4.398) = 11.78$; $p < 0.001$) and explained 11% of the dependent variable variance. Hostile customer behaviors were associated with

TABLE 2.2

Estimation of Emotional Labor Indirect Effects in the Relationship between Disproportionate Customer Expectations and Disengagement from Work ($N = 403$)

Indirect effects B (BootSE)		95% Boot CI	
		BootLLCI	BootULCI
Total	0.004 (0.02)	−0.03	0.04
Disproportionate customer expectations → Deep acting → Disengagement from work	−0.02 (0.01)	−0.04	0.003
Disproportionate customer expectations → Hiding feelings → Disengagement from work	−0.02 (0.02)	−0.07	0.01
Disproportionate customer expectations → Faking emotions → Disengagement from work	0.05 (0.0)	0.02	0.08

Note: B = standardized indirect effect; BootSE = bootstrapped standard error; Boot CI = bootstrapped confidence interval; BootLLCI = bootstrapped lower limit of the confidence interval; BootULCI = bootstrapped upper limit of the confidence interval; level of confidence for the confidence intervals = 95%
***$p < 0.001$. **$p < 0.01$. *$p < 0.05$

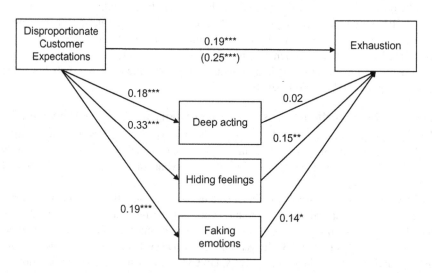

FIGURE 2.2 Regression coefficients of the relationship between disproportionate customer expectations and worker exhaustion, mediated by emotional labor. ***$p < 0.001$. **$p < 0.01$. *$p < 0.05$.

a higher level of disengagement from work, which confirmed hypothesis 1. Hostile customer behaviors were also positively associated with all the analyzed types of emotional labor, which partially confirmed hypothesis 2.

After the introduction of the mediators into the model, the relationship between the independent variable and the dependent variable was reinforced. A single,

TABLE 2.3

Estimation of Emotional Labor Indirect Effects in the Relationship between Disproportionate Customer Expectations and Worker Exhaustion (N = 403)

Indirect effects B (BootSE)		95% Boot CI	
		BootLLCI	**BootULCI**
Total	0.08 (0.02)	0.04	0.12
Disproportionate customer expectations → Deep acting → Exhaustion	0.003 (0.01)	−0.02	0.03
Disproportionate customer expectations → Hiding feelings → Exhaustion	0.05 (0.02)	0.01	0.09
Disproportionate customer expectations → Faking emotions → Exhaustion	0.03 (0.01)	0.004	0.05

Note: B = standardized indirect effect; BootSE = bootstrapped standard error; Boot CI = bootstrapped confidence interval; BootLLCI = bootstrapped lower limit of the confidence interval; BootULCI = bootstrapped upper limit of the confidence interval; level of confidence for the confidence intervals = 95%

significant indirect effect was observed (Table 2.4), which means that a significant indirect effect developed [Hayes 2017]. The relationship between hostile customer behaviors and employee disengagement from work was explained by faking emotions – an aspect of surface acting (Figure 2.3). This result partially confirmed hypothesis 3b, but instead of the assumed mediation mechanism, a mechanism of suppression was observed. However, hypothesis 3a was not confirmed.

TABLE 2.4

Estimation of the Emotional Labor Indirect Effects in the Relationship between Hostile Customer Behaviors and Employee Disengagement from Work (N = 403)

Indirect effects B (BootSE)		95% Boot CI	
		BootLLCI	**BootULCI**
Total	0.01 (0.02)	−0.02	0.05
Hostile customer behaviors → Deep acting → Disengagement from work	−0.01 (0.01)	−0.03	0.004
Hostile customer behaviors → Hiding feelings → Disengagement from work	−0.02 (0.02)	−0.06	0.01
Hostile customer behaviors → Faking emotions → Disengagement from work	0.04 (0.02)	0.02	0.08

Note: B = standardized indirect effect; BootSE = bootstrapped standard error; Boot CI = bootstrapped confidence interval; BootLLCI = bootstrapped lower limit of the confidence interval; BootULCI = bootstrapped upper limit of the confidence interval; level of confidence for the confidence intervals = 95%

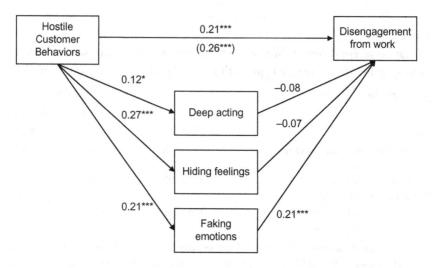

FIGURE 2.3 Regression coefficients of the relationship between hostile customer behaviors and disengagement from work, mediated by emotional labor. ***$p < 0.001$. **$p < 0.01$. *$p < 0.05$.

2.3.1.4 Hostile Customer Behaviors and Worker Exhaustion

The tested model had a good data fit ($F(4.398) = 23.85$; $p < 0.001$) and explained 19% of the dependent variable variance. The relationship between hostile customer behaviors and worker exhaustion was significant and positive, which confirmed hypothesis 1 (Figure 2.4).

Again, the direct association between the independent variable and the dependent variable was reinforced after the introduction of the mediators into the model. A

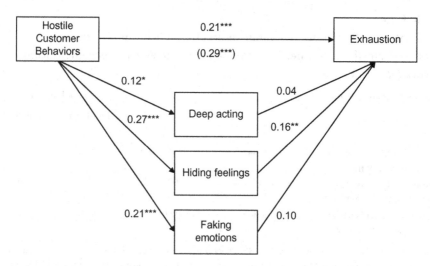

FIGURE 2.4 Regression coefficients of the relationship between hostile customer behaviors and worker exhaustion, mediated by emotional labor. ***$p < 0.001$. **$p < 0.01$. *$p < 0.05$.

TABLE 2.5

Estimation of Emotional Labor Indirect Effects in the Relationship between Hostile Customer Behaviors and Worker Exhaustion (N = 403)

Indirect effects B (BootSE)		95% Boot CI	
		BootLLCI	**BootULCI**
Total	0.07 (0.02)	0.03	0.11
Hostile customer behaviors → Deep acting → Exhaustion	0.005 (0.008)	–0.01	0.02
Hostile customer behaviors → Hiding feelings → Exhaustion	0.04 (0.02)	0.01	0.08
Hostile customer behaviors → Faking emotions → Exhaustion	0.02 (0.01)	0.00	0.05

Note: B = standardized indirect effect; BootSE = bootstrapped standard error; Boot CI = bootstrapped confidence interval; BootLLCI = bootstrapped lower limit of the confidence interval; BootULCI = bootstrapped upper limit of the confidence interval; level of confidence for the confidence intervals = 95%

significant indirect effect was also observed (Table 2.5), which means that a mechanism of suppression could be identified [Hayes 2017]. Hostile customer behaviors have been associated with greater emotional exhaustion among workers, which has partly been explained by hiding feelings – an aspect of surface acting. This result has partially supported hypothesis 3b, but instead of the assumed mediation mechanism, a mechanism of suppression has been observed. Hypothesis 3a has not been confirmed yet again.

2.3.2 THE MEDIATING ROLE OF EMOTIONAL LABOR IN THE RELATIONSHIP BETWEEN STRESS-INDUCING CUSTOMER BEHAVIORS AND THE PHYSICAL WELLBEING OF WORKERS

2.3.2.1 Disproportionate Customer Expectations and the Physical Wellbeing of Workers

The tested model fit the data ($F(4.398)$ = 7.30; $p < 0.001$) and explained 7% of the dependent variable variance. Disproportionate customer expectations were negatively associated with the physical wellbeing of workers, confirming hypothesis 1. The direct relationship between disproportionate customer expectations and the physical wellbeing of workers was mitigated after the introduction of the mediators into the models, but remained significant (Figure 2.5).

The indirect effects analysis (Table 2.6) showed that deep acting and hiding feelings played the role of partial mediators in the relationship between disproportionate customer expectations and the physical wellbeing of workers. This indicates that disproportionate customer expectations have been negatively associated with physical wellbeing, and this relationship has been partly explained by deep acting and hiding feelings. The faking emotions factor was not associated with the physical wellbeing of workers. This result has partially confirmed hypotheses 4a and 4b.

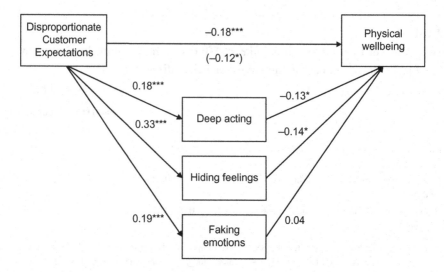

FIGURE 2.5 Regression coefficients of the relationship between disproportionate customer expectations and the physical wellbeing, mediated by emotional labor. ***$p < 0.001$. **$p < 0.01$. *$p < 0.05$.

TABLE 2.6

Estimation of Emotional Labor Indirect Effects in the Relationship between Disproportionate Customer Expectations and the Physical Wellbeing of Workers ($N = 403$)

Indirect effects B (BootSE)		95% Boot CI	
		BootLLCI	BootULCI
Total	−0.06 (0.02)	−0.11	−0.02
Disproportionate customer expectations → Deep acting → Physical wellbeing	−0.02 (0.01)	−0.05	−0.001
Disproportionate customer expectations → Hiding feelings → Physical wellbeing	−0.04 (0.02)	−0.09	−0.01
Excessive demands → Faking emotions → Physical wellbeing	0.01 (0.01)	−0.02	0.03

Note: B = standardized indirect effect; BootSE = bootstrapped standard error; Boot CI = bootstrapped confidence interval; BootLLCI = bootstrapped lower limit of the confidence interval; BootULCI = bootstrapped upper limit of the confidence interval; level of confidence for the confidence intervals = 95%

2.3.2.2 Hostile Customer Behaviors and the Physical Wellbeing of Workers

The tested model fit the data ($F(4.398) = 8.01$; $p < 0.001$) and explained 8% of the dependent variable variance (Table 2.7). Hostile customer behaviors were negatively associated with the physical wellbeing of workers, which confirmed hypothesis 1. The direct relationship between hostile customer behaviors and the physical

TABLE 2.7

Estimation of Emotional Labor Indirect Effects in Relationship between Hostile Customer Behaviors and the Physical Wellbeing of Workers ($N = 403$)

Indirect effects B (BootSE)		95% Boot CI	
		BootLLCI	**BootULCI**
Total	−0.04 (0.02)	−0.09	−0.01
Disproportionate customer expectations → Deep acting → Physical wellbeing	−0.02 (0.01)	−0.04	−0.0001
Disproportionate customer expectations → Hiding feelings → Physical wellbeing	−0.04 (0.02)	−0.08	−0.01
Disproportionate customer expectations → Faking emotions → Physical wellbeing	0.01 (0.01)	−0.01	0.04

Note: B = standardized indirect effect; BootSE = bootstrapped standard error; Boot CI = bootstrapped confidence interval; BootLLCI = bootstrapped lower limit of the confidence interval; BootULCI = bootstrapped upper limit of the confidence interval; level of confidence for the confidence intervals = 95%

wellbeing of workers was weakened after the introduction of the mediators into the models, but remained significant (Figure 2.6).

Two indirect effects were observed. Deep acting and the hiding of feelings partly mediated the relationship between hostile customer behaviors and the physical wellbeing of workers. The indirect effect of deep acting was not strong; however, it was significant. This result has partially supported hypotheses 4a and 4b.

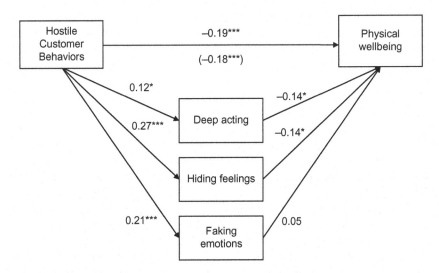

FIGURE 2.6 Regression coefficients of the relationship between hostile customer behaviors and worker physical wellbeing, mediated by emotional labor. ***$p < 0.001$. **$p < 0.01$. *$p < 0.05$.

2.4   SUMMARY AND DISCUSSION OF RESULTS

The conducted study has revealed that stress-inducing customer behaviors are associated with job burnout symptoms and the physical wellbeing of workers: the more frequent the experience of disproportionate customer expectations and hostile customer behaviors, the greater the exhaustion and disengagement from work, and the poorer the physical wellbeing of workers. These results are consistent with previous, albeit limited research findings: customer incivility has been found associated with turnover intention, psychological tension, reduced job satisfaction [Wilson and Holmvall 2013], stress [Sliter et al. 2010; Adams and Webster 2013; Hur, Moon, and Jung 2015], emotional exhaustion [Kern and Grandey 2009; Sliter et al. 2010], reduced motivation to work, poorer creativity [Hur, Moon, and Jung 2015], and a declined psychological wellbeing [Arnold et al. 2015]. So far, there has been a paucity of research into the relationship between stress-inducing customer behaviors and the physical health of workers. An example is a study on the relationship between hostile customer behaviors and sickness absence [Sliter, Sliter, and Jex 2012], or another on the relationship between customer aggression (both verbal and physical) and employee physical health complaints [Dupré, Dawe, and Barling 2014]. The present study offers further evidence for the negative relationship between stress-inducing customer behaviors and job burnout, as well as the less frequently analyzed physical symptoms reported by workers.

The effects of emotional labor have been analyzed mainly in terms of job burnout and job satisfaction so far, and to a lesser extent in the context of physical health. In a study conducted by Lee [2016], the researcher analyzed the prevalence of physical diseases among various occupations, defined in the research as the "Emotional labor job" category, taking the perspective of the "job-focused emotional labor" coined by Brotheridge [2002b]. The research showed that persons employed in emotional labor high-risk jobs were more likely to complain about headaches, abdominal pains, dyspnea, chest pain, fatigue, musculoskeletal pain and other digestive disorders, such as gastritis or irritable bowel syndrome [Lee 2016]. However, it is not known which emotional labor strategies were used by the cited study participants.

The present research has shown that deep acting emotional labor and hiding feelings have been associated with poorer physical health, mediating the relationship between stress-inducing customer behaviors and the physical health of workers. Until now, there have been observed rather positive effects of deep acting on job satisfaction, or personal accomplishment [Brotheridge 2002b; Zhang and Zhu 2008], while negative effects have been relatively rare [e.g. Mann and Cowburn 2005], or not identified at all [e.g. Grandey 2003; Näring, Briët, and Brouwers 2007]. Similarly, the present study results have not shown any relationship between deep acting and job burnout of workers. However, the study results have revealed that significant associations occur at the level of physical wellbeing. It seems that the effort associated with emotional regulation undertaken by the workers exposed to stress-inducing customer behaviors translates into physical symptoms such as: accelerated heart rate, stomach ailments, weakness, chest tightness, or sleeping problems. Customer service workers who produce deep acting emotional labor have greater job satisfaction and a sense of accomplishment, and their customers are also more satisfied with the provided service [e.g. Brotheridge 2002b; Grandey 2003]. This may explain why such workers are less affected by job burnout. However, handling difficult customers with the deep emotional labor strategy continues to drain the worker's resources and energy, resulting in physical symptoms. According to the Conservation of Resource Theory [Hobfoll 1989], the effort invested in emotional labor should be rewarded to replenish the depleted resources [Brotheridge 2002a]. Perhaps customer satisfaction or confidence in good performance and self-accomplishment are not sufficient to reward the losses incurred as a result of exposure to hostile customer behaviors or disproportionate customer expectations.

The relationship between surface acting emotional labor and job burnout has already been investigated by previous research [Brotheridge 2002b], and it has been supported by the present study's evidence. Nevertheless, the current research has been one of the very few accounts of the proven mediating role of emotional labor in the relationship between stress-inducing customer behavior and job burnout, and physical wellbeing.

At the same time, the models explaining physical wellbeing and one of the aspects of job burnout – disengagement from work – have been characterized in the present study by a lower degree of the explained variance than those explaining the level of worker exhaustion (the second aspect of job burnout). The physical wellbeing and disengagement from work level variance was explained in the mediation models within a 7–11% range (depending on the model variables), while the exhaustion variance was explained within a 17–20% range. This suggests that exhaustion is most strongly associated with stress-inducing customer behaviors and the emotional labor performed by workers. Perhaps exhaustion is the first in a series of symptoms: effects on the level of physical wellbeing, or reduced work engagement. One part of the relationship (where physical wellbeing was a dependent variable) was also found to explain the mechanism of partial mediation, while the other part (where job burnout was a dependent variable) explained the mechanism of suppression; this means that the mediating variables reinforced the relationship between stress-inducing customer behaviors and worker exhaustion, or disengagement from work. In some cases, however, there were minor alterations in the strength of the relationship between the independent and dependent variables. It therefore seems that other variables or models, not included in the present study, may be responsible for these relationships.

Until present, most studies of emotional labor have been focused on its effects as an independent variable. Equally, the problem of stressful/unpleasant behavior at work, or 'incivility', has been studied much more often in the context of co-worker or management behaviors rather than customer behaviors [Schilpzand, Pater, and Erez 2014]. Similar results were reported by Adams and Webster [2013], whereby surface acting emotional labor partially mediated the relationship between customer incivility and work-related stress among workers.

The novelty of the present research is in the analysis of surface acting distinguished into two aspects – faking emotions and hiding feelings – which has revealed the different roles of each aspect. Hiding feelings was found to be negatively associated with the physical wellbeing of workers, while the faking-emotions factor was not significantly associated with this variable. Hiding feelings was also related with exhaustion stronger than faking emotions. In turn, hiding feelings was not associated with disengagement from work, whereas faking emotions was related to a lower job engagement. However, both types of the stress-inducing customer behavior (disproportionate customer expectations and hostile customer behaviors) were most strongly related to faking emotions.

Contrary to hypothesis 2, stress-inducing customer behavior was positively related to deep acting. This suggests that even in emotionally difficult situations, workers use all forms of emotional labor. Grandey, Dickter and Sin [2004] showed that employees who felt threatened when faced with customer aggression used the surface acting strategy, while those who did not feel threatened used deep acting. Therefore, individual risk assessment may be important.

2.4.1 STRENGTHS AND LIMITATIONS

In the present research, the rarely analyzed relationship between stress-inducing customer behaviors, emotional labor and physical symptoms has been investigated. Also analyzed was the effect of emotional labor strategies in the context of stressful, hostile customer behaviors, which might help to improve understanding of these phenomena, usually studied separately. Although the study was conducted in a group of tax administration workers – rare participants in this kind of research – most respondents were women, which may be a limitation of the study. Women use the deep acting strategy more often than men [Schaubroeck and Jones 2000], thus further research should consider the possibility of comparing both genders and different sectors. The presented statistical analyses were carried out using cross-sectional study data, therefore the conclusions should be treated with caution, particularly those concerning mediation/suppression analyses. It should be noted that some of the tested models did not show strong relationships, thus, it is worth looking at other variables that may be relevant in the described relationships, as well as other ways to explain them, and greater caution should be taken with the results of this study. The role of resources that help workers cope with these types of stressors has also not been considered in the study – such a topic is thus worth exploring in further research.

2.5 CONCLUSIONS

The study suggests that in stress-inducing customer behavior working conditions, workers who fake emotions incur the lowest personal costs, unlike employees who use deep acting emotional labor and those who hide feelings. However, faking emotions as a form of coping with hostile customer behaviors has been found most strongly associated with disengagement from work. Further research should identify individual and organizational resources that help workers cope with such social stressors and develop effective interventions to provide employees with coping resources.

REFERENCES

Adams, G. A., and J. R. Webster. 2013. Emotional regulation as a mediator between interpersonal mistreatment and distress. *Eur J Work Organ Psychol* 22(6):697–710.

Arnold, K. A., C. E. Connelly, M. M. Walsh, and K. A. Martin Ginis. 2015. Leadership styles, emotion regulation, and burnout. *J Occup Health Psychol* 20(4):481.

Baka, L. 2015. Does job burnout mediate negative effects of job demands on mental and physical health in a group of teachers? Testing the energetic process of job demands-resources model. *Int J Occup Environ Med* 28(2):335.

Bazińska, D., and D. Szczygieł. 2012. Doświadczane emocje i ich regulacja jako wyznaczniki wypalenia zawodowego pracowników usług. *Czasopismo Psychologiczne* 18:119–130.

Brotheridge, C. M., and R. T. Lee. 2002. Testing a conservation of resources model of the dynamics of emotional labor. *J Occup Health Psychol* 7(1):57–67.

Brotheridge, C. M., and A. A. Grandey. 2002. Emotional Labour and burnout: Comparing two perspectives of "people work". *J Vocat Behav* 60(1):17–39.

Brotheridge, C. M., and R. T. Lee. 2003. Development and validation of the Emotional Labor Scale. *J Occup Organ Psychol* 76:365–379.

Cieślak, R., and M. Widerszal-Bazyl. 2000. *Psychospołeczne warunki pracy: Podręcznik do kwestionariusza [The Psychosocial Working Conditions Questionnaire].* Warszawa: CIOP-PIB.

Demerouti, E., A. B. Bakker, I. Vardakou, and A. Kantas. 2003. The convergent validity of two burnout instruments: A multitrait-multimethod analysis. *Eur J Psychol Assess* 19(1):12.

Dormann, C., and D. Zapf. 2004. Customer-related social stressors and burnout. *J Occup Health Psychol* 9(1):61–82.

Dupré, K. E., K. A. Dawe, and J. Barling. 2014. Harm to those who serve: Effects of direct and vicarious customer-initiated workplace aggression. *J Interpers Violence* 29(13):2355–2377.

Finogenow, M., M. Wróbel, and J. Mróz. 2015. Skala płytkiej i głębokiej pracy emocjonalnej (SPGPE) – adaptacja narzędzia i analiza własności psychometrycznych. [Deep Acting and Surface Acting Scale (DASAS) – Adaptation of the metod and preliminary psychometric properties]. *Med Pr* 66(3):359–371. doi: 10.13075/mp.5893.00168.

Gountas, S., J. Gountas, G. Soutar, and F. Mavondo. 2014. Delivering good service: Personal resources, job satisfaction and nurses' 'customer' (patient) orientation. *J Adv Nurs* 70(7):1553–1563.

Grandey, A. A., A. P. Tam, and A. L. Brauburger. 2002. Affective states and traits in the workplace: Diary and survey data from young workers. *Motiv Emot* 26:31–55.

Grandey, A. A. 2003. When "the show must go on": Surface acting and deep acting as determinants of emotional exhaustion and peer-rated service delivery. *Acad Manag J* 46(1):86–96.

Grandey, A. A., D. N. Dickter, and H. Sin. 2004. The customer is not always right: Customer aggression and emotion regulation of service employees. *J Organ Behav* 25(3):397–418.

Grandey, A. A., G. M. Fisk, A. S. Mattila, K. J. Jansen, and L. A. Sideman. 2005. Is "service with a smile" enough? Authenticity of positive displays during service encounters. *Organ Behav Hum Decis Process* 96(1):38–55.

Gross, J. 1998. Antecedent- and response-focused emotion regulation: divergent consequences for experience,expression, and physiology. *Journal of Personality and Social Psychology*, 74:224–237.

GUS [Główny Urząd Statystyczny]. 2014. *Accidents at Work and Work-Related Health Problems. Statistical Information and Elaborations.* Warszawa: Główny Urząd Statystyczny. https://stat.gov.pl/obszary-tematyczne/rynek-pracy/warunki-pracy-wypadki-przy-pracy/wypadki-przy-pracy-i-problemy-zdrowotne-zwiazane-z-praca,2,2.html (accessed January 28, 2020).

Han, S. J., M. A. Bonn, and M. Cho. 2016. The relationship between customer incivility, restaurant frontline service employee burnout and turnover intention. *Int J Hosp Manag* 52:97–106.

Hayes, A. F. 2017. *Introduction to Mediation, Moderation, and Conditional Process Analysis: A Regression-Based Approach.* New York: Guilford Publications.

Hobfoll, S. E. 1989. Conservation of resources: A new attempt at conceptualizing stress. *American Psychol* 44(3):513.

Hochschild, A. R. 1983. *The Managed Heart: Commercialization of Human Feeling.* Berkeley, CA: University of California Press.

Hur, W. M., T. W. Moon, and Y. S. Jung. 2015. Customer response to employee emotional labor: The structural relationship between emotional labor, job satisfaction, and customer satisfaction. *J Serv Mark* 29(1):71–80.

Kern, J. H., and A. A. Grandey. 2009. Customer incivility as a social stressor: The role of race and racial identity for service employees. *J Occup Health Psychol* 14(1):46–57. doi: 10.1037/a0012684.

Kong, H., and J. E. Jeon. 2018. Daily emotional labor, negative affect state, and emotional exhaustion: Cross-level moderators of affective commitment. *Sustainability* 10(6):1967.

Lee, R. T., B. L. Lovell, and C. M. Brotheridge. 2010. Tenderness and steadiness: Relating job and interpersonal demands and resources with burnout and physical symptoms of stress in Canadian physicians. *J Appl Soc Psychol* 40(9):2319–2342.

Lee, S. 2016. P241 Does the emotional labour affect health? The current status of emotional labour and the association with physical health among workers dealing with clients in Korea. *Occup Environ Med* 73(1):A202.

Mann, S., and J. Cowburn. 2005. Emotional labour and stress within mental health nursing. *J Psychiatr Ment Health Nurs* 12:154–162.

Näring, G., M. Briët, and A. Brouwers. 2007. Validation of the Dutch questionnaire on emotional labor (D-QEL) in nurses and teachers. *Psychosoc Resour Hum Serv Work* 21(39):135–145.

Parent-Thirion, A., Biletta, I., Cabrita, J., Vargas, O., Vermeylen, G., Wilczyńska, A., and Wilkens, M. 2017. Sixth European Working Conditions Survey: Overview report (2017 update). Luxembourg: Publications Office of the European Union. www.eurofound.europa.eu/publications/report/2016/working-conditions/sixth-european-working-conditions-survey-overview-report (accessed January 28, 2020).

Rathi, N., D. Bhatnagar, and S. K. Mishra. 2013. Effect of emotional labor on emotional exhaustion and work attitudes among hospitality employees in India. *J Hum Resour Hosp Tour* 12(3):273–290.

Schaubroeck, J., and J. R. Jones. 2000. Antecedents of workplace emotional labor dimensions and moderators of their effects on physical symptoms. *J Organ Behav* 21(2):163–183.

Schilpzand, P., I. E. De Pater, and A. Erez. 2014. Workplace incivility: A review of the literature and agenda for future research. *J Organ Behav* 37(Suppl 1):s57–s88.

Singh, J., J. R. Goolsby, and G. K. Rhoads. 1994. Behavioral and psychological consequences of boundary spanning burnout for customer service representatives. *J Mark Res* 31(4):558–569.

Sliter, M., S. Jex, K. Wolford, and J. McInnerney. 2010. How rude! Emotional labor as a mediator between customer incivility and employee outcomes. *J Occup Health Psychol* 15(4):468–481. doi: 10.1037/a0020723.

Sliter, M., K. Sliter, and S. Jex. 2012. The employee as a punching bag: The effect of multiple sources of incivility on employee withdrawal behavior and sales performance. *J Organ Behav* 33(1):121–139.

Szczygieł, D., R. Bazińska, R. Kadzikowska-Wrzosek, and S. Retowski. 2009. Praca emocjonalna w zawodach usługowych: Pojęcie, przegląd teorii i badań. *Psychologia Społeczna* 4(3):155–166.

Szczygieł, D., and R. Bazińska. 2013. *The Stress-Inducing Customer Behavior Scale –* Trudny klient jako źródło stresu w pracy usługowej. Konstrukcja i psychometryczne właściwości Skali Stresujących Zachowań Klienta (SSZK). *Czasopismo Psychologiczne* 19:227–239.

van Jaarsveld, D. D., D. D. Walker, and D. P. Skarlicki. 2010. The role of job demands and emotional exhaustion in the relationship between customer and employee incivility. *J Manag* 36(6):1486–1504.

Wilson, N. L., and C. M. Holmvall. 2013. The development and validation of the incivility from customers scale. *J Occup Health Psychol* 18(3):310.

Zammuner, V. L., and C. Galli. 2005. Wellbeing: Causes and consequences of emotion regulation in work settings. *Int Rev Psychiatry* 17(5):355–364.

Zapf, D., A. Isic, M. Bechtoldt, and P. Blau. 2003. What is typical for call centre jobs? Job characteristics, and service interactions in different call centres. *Eur J Work Organ Psychol* 12(4):311–340.

Zhang, Q., and W. Zhu. 2008. Exploring emotion in teaching: Emotional labor, burnout, and satisfaction in Chinese higher education. *Commun Educ* 57(1):105–122.

3 The Relationship between Intensification of Stress-Inducing Customer Behaviors, Job Burnout, and Well-Being of Customer Service Workers
The Role of Emotional Labor Types

Andrzej Najmiec

CONTENTS

3.1 INTRODUCTION

The causes of work-related stress may be related both to job demands resulting from
the specificity of the profession and the workplace – e.g. tasks performed, physical
working environment, direct customer service interactions, and psychosocial working conditions specific to the social and organizational environment.

A particular manifestation of prolonged stress at work is the phenomenon of job
burnout. Job burnout occurs mainly in professions related to the provision of direct
services/assistance to other persons, including working with patients, customers, students, etc.

Stress experienced by employees affects the functioning of the entire organization and is reflected in such organizational aspects as increased absenteeism, increased costs associated with a higher morbidity, reduced productivity, increased number of accidents, higher staff turnover, hostile working atmosphere, or increased likelihood of workplace bullying. Identifying the causes of workplace stress is the first step in reducing its levels. The next step is to take action to prevent negative health effects.

3.2   CUSTOMER SERVICE WORK AND STRESS RESEARCH

Customer social relations and the resulting specificity of stressors depend on the characteristics of work performed by different occupational groups. The diversity of these conditions has been demonstrated by numerous studies. A theoretical discussion of the research related to stress-inducing customer behaviors and emotional labor can be found in Chapter 2.

A particular type of customer service work is performed by civil servants, whose duties include receiving applications and handling official matters, often of high personal importance to the applicants (e.g. applications for various types of social security entitlements). Perhaps this is the reason for the very high levels of occupational stress observed in this professional group in Europe, just after healthcare workers [Milczarek, Schneider, and Gonzales 2009].

3.3   JOB BURNOUT

Customer service work is often associated with the phenomenon of job burnout. Job burnout is a response to prolonged stress, which is particularly common in occupations involving direct customer/patient/beneficiary contacts.

The most widely used concept of job burnout defines the phenomenon as a psychological set of three symptoms:

- emotional exhaustion – feelings of excessive emotional burden and depletion of individual emotional resources, mainly caused by excessive job demands,
- depersonalization – lack of empathy and indifference in relation to other people, who are usually the service/assistance/care recipients,
- reduced perception of personal achievements – a decreased confidence in personal competences and achievements, mainly associated with the working environment [Maslach, Schaufeli, and Leiter 2001].

Initially, the phenomenon of job burnout was considered as related only to social services workers (e.g. doctors, nursing home workers, teachers). Later studies showed that similar signs of job burnout also occur in non-aid professions, such as managers, sales representatives, or IT specialists [Demerouti et al. 2001], i.e. other professions involving frequent interaction with customers/clients. In response to such research findings, Maslach and Leiter [2008] proposed a new definition of job burnout so that the research could be extended to other professions. The components of job burnout have thus been redefined:

- depersonalization has been replaced by the term *cynicism*, which refers not only to a distanced attitude toward people but also to the entire working environment,
- reduced perception of personal achievements has been narrowed down to a sense of lack of professional achievements,
- emotional exhaustion has been replaced by the term *exhaustion*, meaning not only a decreased vitality but also a loss of physical strength [Maslach and Leiter 2008].

Another standard approach to the phenomenon of job burnout has been introduced by the authors of the *job demands–resources* model [Demerouti et al. 2001]. The researchers define job burnout as a long-term effect of occupational stress caused by excessive job demands, whereby stress levels can be regulated by the personal resources of workers. In this sense, job burnout comprises two components: exhaustion and disengagement from work. The latter has been used by Demerouti et al. [2001] to replace *depersonalization* as an emotional withdrawal in direct customer service work. Disengagement from work has been here defined as a distanced attitude toward customers, co-workers and the entire working environment, e.g. duties, organizational values, or culture. Disengagement from work is therefore a broader term and includes both depersonalization and lack of personal achievements. According to the authors, the same working environment factors that induce the stress response contribute to the development of job burnout; however, job burnout develops over a longer period than stress.

Research suggests that the main cause of job burnout is work-related stress. The stress factors include excessive workload, low job control, conflict of values, time pressure, difficult interpersonal relationships, or high emotional demands.

The relationship between the above-mentioned factors and job burnout has been confirmed in empirical studies conducted in various professional groups. Most of the research has shown that the workload correlates positively with all the dimensions of job burnout [Demerouti et al. 2001]. Also, the relationship between job control and job burnout has been proven by many researchers. Jawahar, Stone, and Kisamore [2007], in their study on IT specialists, examined the relationship between role conflict and job burnout. They showed that workers experiencing a stronger role conflict in the organization had a higher job burnout rate compared to workers declaring a lesser role conflict.

Job burnout syndrome affects the physical and mental health of workers. It is associated with poor job satisfaction, declining performance, deterioration of private life, growing somatic complaints and other health problems, a pessimistic approach to life, depression, and anxiety disorders. The consequences of job burnout also affect organizations, contributing to absenteeism, increased staff turnover, lower productivity, deteriorating relations between co-workers, surging sickness absence, and employee medical treatment costs, or the costs of hiring new employees [Ostrowska and Michcik 2013].

Also in the Polish research, the problem of job burnout has been discussed. The research aimed at adapting the Polish version of the Oldenburg Occupational Exposure Questionnaire (the OLBI tool, developed by Demerouti et al. [2001]) has shown that burnout (exhaustion and disengagement from work) is associated with stress and work engagement. The higher the level of job burnout observed among the surveyed professional services and social services workers, the greater the experienced stress at work, and the lesser the work engagement of those workers who declared reduced vitality and a lower level of work engagement and absorption by work tasks [Baka and Basińska 2016].

A review article on emotional labor and burnout by Jeung, Kim, and Chang [2018] covered almost 100 publications on the problem of burnout, the consequences of emotional labor, and the relationship between emotional labor and burnout, taking into account the work environment and individual characteristics of workers. Part of the research is related to the impact of individual employee variables on job burnout. Important features included: self-efficacy, individual perception of one's own social capital, and Type A behavior pattern (TABP).

High emotional demands contributing to job burnout of workers have been recognized by experts as a particular occupational risk in the changing world of work. Workers may try to suppress the difficulties in coping with these demands for fear of losing their job, which effectively is a source of stress. According to EU-OSHA experts [Milczarek and Brun 2007], this problem may particularly affect the professional services and healthcare sectors. An important factor raising the emotional job demands is workplace bullying, identified as one of the major stress factors, affecting mental and physical health of workers. It can be practiced by managers, co-workers and customers alike.

A high rate of workplace bullying, i.e. 6.9–7.4% [GUS 2014], recorded among public administration (including social insurance) workers suggest that these sector workers are more exposed to stress-inducing customer interactions, or higher emotional job demands. Emotional demands are associated with a phenomenon which has been defined as *emotional labor.*

3.4 EMOTIONAL LABOR

Emotional labor has been defined in various ways. The term *job-focused emotional labor* describes the level of emotional job demands specific to a profession. This approach has been often used in research on customer service occupations, where such demands as frequency of customer contact or expectations related to expressing emotions are measured [Brotheridge and Grandey 2002]. The second approach to emotional labor constitutes the concept of *employee-focused emotional labor* which relates to regulating and expressing emotions in compliance with the employer-set standards, aiming to meet the job demands. In this approach, the emotional dissonance that occurs when a worker expresses feelings other than those actually felt, and the processes of regulating the employee expressed emotions to fulfill the job demands, are measured [Brotheridge and Lee 2002].

Hochschild [1983] has identified two distinct types of employee-focused emotional labor: surface acting and deep acting. The definitions of surface and deep acting can be found in Chapter 2, this volume.

Hochschild [1983] distinguishes six groups of occupations that place emotional job demands on workers: freelance professions (e.g. lawyers and doctors), managers and administration staff, sales assistants and other sales/retail professions, civil servants, household workers, and other non-household services, e.g. hospitality, restaurant or beauty professions.

Szczygieł et al. [2009] generalized the above category list into two occupational groups involving emotional labor demands: commercial occupations (e.g. waiters, salesmen) and social service occupations (e.g. nurses, teachers). Emotional labor intensifies as the number of direct customer contacts grows.

3.5 THE CULTURAL EFFECTS OF EMOTIONAL LABOR

The consequences of emotional labor also depend on cultural differences. Allen, Diefendorff, and Ma [2014] analyzed the emotional labor of professional services sector workers in the United States and China. The study results showed that in the case of Chinese workers, the relationship between surface acting and job burnout was weaker than in the group of American workers. In the latter employee group, the emotional regulation resulted in surface acting, whereas this relationship was reversed among the Chinese workers – emotional regulation was associated with a lower intensity of surface acting. These results show that the study of emotional labor should also take into account the cultural context.

3.6 INDIVIDUAL FACTORS AND EFFECTS OF EMOTIONAL LABOR

The phenomenon of emotional labor has recently been the subject of Polish research. In research by Wróbel [2013], the author presented results of a study conducted in a group of teachers. The aim of the study was to analyze the relationship between emotional labor and job burnout of teachers, taking into account the role of emotional intelligence. The study accounted for the role of personal resources in coping with the effects of emotional labor, particularly given that the tendency to use emotional labor (surface or deep acting) may depend on various individual and situational factors [Brotheridge 2006]. Individual factors include gender, emotional expressiveness, positive and negative affectivity, and emotional intelligence. According to researchers, the latter is positively associated with deep acting and negatively associated with surface acting [Austin, Dore, and O'Donovan 2008; Brotheridge 2006]. However, other research has shown that the effectiveness of influencing customer reactions is greater when the emotions displayed by the employee are authentic [Grandey et al. 2005; Hennig-Thurau et al. 2006]. Statistical analyses conducted in the study in the teacher group showed that the relationship between emotional labor (surface acting and deep acting) and job burnout was significant. The results also proved that emotional intelligence moderated these relationships. In the high emotional intelligence study group, the relationship between surface acting and emotional exhaustion, depersonalization, and a lower sense of personal accomplishment vanished. In the high emotional intelligence study group, the relationship between deep acting, emotional exhaustion, and depersonalization was insignificant. This suggests that a high level of emotional intelligence mitigates the negative effects of emotional labor, i.e. the symptoms of job burnout [Wróbel 2013].

In a study by Szczygieł and Bazińska [2013] in the group of service sector employees, the author revealed that negative affect was significantly associated with a higher level of emotional exhaustion, while high positive affect showed an inverse association. It was found that workers declaring higher intensity of negative emotions reported more symptoms of emotional exhaustion. However, this was observed only in the group of workers with a low level of emotional intelligence.

Also, in research conducted by Sliter et al. [2013], the role of emotional intelligence in the work of professional services sector employees was analyzed. In addition, another individual factor was taken into account, i.e. the age of the employees. The results showed that the older the employees were, the more often they used deep acting to the detriment of surface acting.

In search of other individual factors that could be related to the effects of emotional labor, Maneotis, Grandey, and Krauss [2014] conducted a study in a group of grocery store retail workers. The aim of the study was to examine whether emotional labor influenced the relationship between prosocial motives and work performance. The study did not prove the estimated positive role of deep acting, although persons characterized by a high level of prosocial motives used this form of emotional labor to a greater extent. The study showed that the surface acting strategy enabled persons with a low level of prosocial motives to pretend they wanted to offer help to their customers. In the high prosocial motivation employee study group, a high level of customer service work performance was also observed, but only when the employees restrained from surface acting.

3.7 ORGANIZATIONAL FACTORS AND EFFECTS OF EMOTIONAL LABOR

In search of organizational factors influencing the relationship between emotional labor and its effects (job burnout and satisfaction with life), Gopalan, Culbertson, and Leiva [2012] analyzed in their research the role of job control. The conducted study among university staff showed that the relationship between surface acting and emotional exhaustion was stronger among those employees who declared a low level of job control, which also affected their overall satisfaction with life. However, no such relationships were observed in the case of deep acting.

The results of studies analyzing the consequence (particularly the positive effects) of emotional labor have been ambiguous and require further analyses, which would account for the impact of other variables [Szczygieł et al. 2009]. An example of such a factor can be psychosocial working conditions.

Regarding *job-focused emotional labor*, the theory of emotional labor can be applied to the *job demands-control-support* occupational stress model [Karasek and Theorell 1990; Brotheridge and Grandey 2002]. The job demands refer to the requirements of employee–customer interaction, while the control relates to the ability to regulate emotions expressed at work. Therefore, the emotional labor types have been considered in studies aimed at investigating the relationship between psychosocial working conditions and stress-inducing customer contacts, and job burnout and well-being of employees. The emotional labor variable may enable a more thorough analysis of these relationships. In the present study, the moderating role of emotional labor (surface acting and deep acting) in the relationship between the intensity of stress-inducing customer behavior and the job burnout and well-being of customer service employees has been examined using a combined regression and interaction analysis.

3.8 STUDY GROUPS

A survey study has been conducted in all 14 voivodships of Poland by a social research agency. The surveyed groups were persons employed in insurance services, i.e. direct customer contact professions, and consisted in social insurance workers ($n = 200$), and employees of private insurance companies ($n = 198$), referred to as private insurance workers (Tables 3.1 and 3.2).

The study has also encompassed the following, other groups of workers: tax administration services, telephone customer service, and health care workers. The obtained results in the group of tax administration workers are presented in Chapter 2.

The average sickness absence in the private insurance employee group had been about six days in the preceding year, while in the group of social insurance workers it had amounted to eight days.

The average time spent working with customers was similar in both groups and amounted to 6.66 hours in the private insurance employee group, and 6.74 hours in the social insurance employee group.

3.9 METHOD

3.9.1 THE PSYCHOSOCIAL WORKING CONDITIONS QUESTIONNAIRE

The Psychosocial Working Conditions Questionnaire [Cieślak and Widerszal-Bazyl 2000], which is based on the *job demands-control-support* occupation stress

TABLE 3.1
Age in the Surveyed Respondent Groups

Workers	Min.	Max.	Mean	Deviation std.
Private insurance	21	66	37.4	9.46
Social insurance	25	66	43.8	8.75

TABLE 3.2
Gender Distribution in the Surveyed Respondent Groups

Workers	Total sample size	Female	Male
Private insurance	198	152	46
Social insurance	200	180	20

model [Karasek and Theorell 1990], was used to measure the psychosocial working conditions.

The questionnaire comprises five theoretical scales and empirical subscales:

- the job demands scale – intellectual, psychophysical, safety responsibilities, role conflict, and workload,
- the job control scale – behavioral, cognitive,
- the social support scale – management and co-worker support,
- the well-being scale – physical and mental well-being,
- the expected changes scale.

The internal consistency index (Cronbach's α) of individual theoretical scales has been high. The job demands scale ranges from Cronbach's $\alpha = 0.74$ to 0.87; the control scale ranges from Cronbach's $\alpha = 0.79$ to 0.86; the social support scale ranges from Cronbach's $\alpha = 0.92$ to 0.96; the well-being scale rangers from Cronbach's $\alpha = 0.88$ to 0.91; and the expected changes scale ranges from Cronbach's $\alpha = 0.88$ to 0.93, for individual occupational groups [Cieślak and Widerszal-Bazyl 2000].

3.9.2 THE STRESS-INDUCING CUSTOMER BEHAVIOR SCALE

The Stress-Inducing Customer Behavior Scale [Szczygieł and Bazińska 2013] was used to measure the intensity of stress-inducing customer behaviors that appear in customer service employee–customer interactions. It consists of 12 items and contains 2 scales:

1. *Hostile customer behavior* (hostile attitudes and negative emotions that customers reveal when interacting with customer service employees), and
2. *Disproportionate customer expectations* (difficult to meet, unclear or excessive, i.e. exceeding standard service, customer expectations).

The reliability and accuracy analysis of the questionnaire has been carried out in a group of professional services employees ($N = 318$). The Cronbach's α reliability ratios for each of the scales have been above 0.80. The scale accuracy tests have shown that the questionnaire results correlate significantly with a higher level of job burnout of workers.

3.9.3 THE OLDENBURG BURNOUT INVENTORY

The Oldenburg Burnout Inventory (OLBI) questionnaire developed by Demerouti et al. [2001] was used for the assessment of job burnout. The Polish version of OLBI [Baka and Basińska 2016] has a two-factor structure that includes exhaustion and disengagement from work. Exhaustion is defined as a result of persistent, chronic tension caused by physical, emotional and cognitive job demands. Disengagement from work relates to a withdrawn attitude toward customers, co-workers, work content and the entire working environment, e.g. tasks, organizational values and culture.

The questionnaire consists of 16 items and contains 2 burnout scales: exhaustion and disengagement from work. Analyses have shown that both exhaustion and disengagement from work are characterized by a satisfactory reliability – Cronbach's α = 0.73 and 0.69, respectively [Baka and Basińska 2016].

3.9.4   DEEP ACTING AND SURFACE ACTING SCALE (DASAS)

The *Deep Acting and Surface Acting Scale (DASAS)* [Finogenow, Wróbel, and Mróz 2015] allows the measurement of the types of emotional labor –deep acting and two aspects of surface acting (hiding feelings and faking emotions). *Surface acting* refers to worker behavior that limits his or her regulatory effort to external emotional expression without interfering with inner feelings. *Deep acting*, in turn, focuses on the emotions felt by the worker (and not on the form of expression). The scale consists of nine items, which are answered on a five-point response scale (from never to always). The internal consistency index (Cronbach's α) of individual scales have been as follows: Cronbach's α = 0.67 for the deep acting subscale; Cronbach's α = 0.80 for the hiding feelings subscale; and Cronbach's α = 0.72 for the faking emotions subscale.

3.10   DESCRIPTIVE STATISTICS

Tables 3.3–3.6 present descriptive statistics of the analyzed job burnout, type of emotional labor, stress-inducing customer behaviors, psychosocial working conditions, and well-being scales in the private insurance and social insurance employee groups.

As far as psychosocial indicators of working conditions are concerned, significant differences were found in the level of behavioral control ($p < 0.001$), cognitive control ($p < 0.001$), perceived social support by both management ($p < 0.001$) and co-workers ($p < 0.001$). Social insurance workers assessed the level of cognitive control higher, whereas behavioral control was assessed lower. In terms of social support, a higher level was recorded in the group of social insurance workers, both in the case of support by managers and by co-workers.

TABLE 3.3

Mean Scores of the Job Burnout Scales – The OLBI Questionnaire Results

Scale	Social insurance workers N = 200		Private insurance workers N = 198	
	Mean	SD	Mean	SD
Disengagement from work	2.22	0.62	2.17	0.46
Exhaustion	2.33*	0.60	2.17	0.52

* p<0.01 (Mann–Whitney Test)

A significant difference between the occupational groups was observed in the level of exhaustion ($p < 0.01$). A higher level of exhaustion was found in the group of social insurance workers.

TABLE 3.4
Mean Scores of the Emotional Labor *Deep Acting and Surface Acting Scale*

Scale/subscale	Social insurance workers N = 200		Private insurance workers N = 198	
	Mean	SD	Mean	SD
Deep acting	2.83	0.78	2.77	0.76
Hiding feelings	3.06*	0.84	2.58	0.83
Faking emotions	2.41	0.76	2.27	0.75

* $p<0.001$ (Mann–Whitney Test)
In terms of emotional labor indicators, a significant difference was observed in hiding feelings ($p < 0.001$). Hiding feelings was more frequent in the group of social insurance workers.

TABLE 3.5
Mean Scores of the *Stress-Inducing Customer Behavior Scale*

Scale	Social insurance workers N = 200		Private insurance workers N = 198	
	Mean	SD	Mean	SD
Hostile customer behaviors	20.14*	6.01	16.64	5.24
Disproportionate customer expectations	22.11*	4.91	19.88	4.40

* $p<0.001$ (Mann–Whitney Test)
Significant differences were observed in both indicators of stress-inducing customer behaviors ($p < 0.001$). Social insurance workers experienced more aggressive behaviors as well as disproportionate customer expectations.

Significant differences were also observed in physical ($p < 0.001$) and mental ($p < 0.001$) well-being. Both well-being indicators were higher in the private insurance employee group.

To answer the question "Does the emotional labor type moderate the relationship between the intensity of stress-inducing customer behavior, the job burnout and well-being of customer service workers?", a series of regression and interaction analyses were conducted with emotional labor (deep acting, faking emotions and hiding feelings) as a moderator. The analyses were conducted using the SPSS 23 Macro Process, Model 1 [Hayes 2013] and O'Connor macros software [1998]. Due to the number of conducted analyses (three moderators, two independent variables, four dependent variables – divided into two analyzed groups of workers), only the significant interactions have been presented.

TABLE 3.6

Mean Scores of the Job Control, Social Support, Well-Being, and Expected Changes Scales – *The Psychosocial Working Conditions Questionnaire* **Results**

Scale/subscale	Social insurance workers N = 200		Private insurance workers N = 198	
	Mean	SD	Mean	SD
Job demands	3.16	0.39	3.21	0.35
Job control	3.29	0.48	3.39	0.41
Social support	3.75*	0.64	3.45	0.73
Well-being	3.61*	0.59	3.88	0.51
Expected changes	2.91	0.83	3.03	0.72
Intellectual demands	3.36	0.53	3.38	0.42
Psychophysical demands and safety responsibilities	3.76	0.52	3.83	0.46
Role conflict and workload demands	2.27	0.57	2.18	0.56
Behavioral control	2.58*	0.62	2.94	0.58
Cognitive control	4.06*	0.49	3.92	0.47
Management support	3.70*	0.81	3.42	0.79
Co-worker support	3.80*	0.64	3.48	0.77
Physical well-being	3.67*	0.66	4.04	0.59
Mental well-being	3.55*	0.59	3.71	0.52

* $p < 0.001$ (Mann–Whitney Test)

3.11 RESULTS

3.11.1 PRIVATE INSURANCE WORKERS

3.11.1.1 The Moderating Role of Deep Acting in the Relationship between the Intensity of Abusive Customer Behavior and the Physical Well-Being of Employees

An interactive component regression analysis showed that the effect of deep acting–hostile customer behaviors interaction was significant in predicting the level of the physical well-being of employees ($b = 0.03$; $p < 0.001$), and the model fit the data.

The workers who performed the greatest deep acting were found, in conditions of frequent, hostile customer behaviors, to be characterized by the poorest physical well-being. In turn, those employees who, despite frequent, hostile customer behaviors, did the lowest levels of the deep acting were found to enjoy the greatest physical well-being.

3.11.1.2 The Moderating Role of Deep Acting in the Relationship between the Intensity of Hostile Customer Behaviors and the Mental Well-Being of Workers

A similar relationship was found in predicting the level of mental well-being. An interactive component regression analysis showed that the deep acting–hostile customer behaviors interaction effect was significant in predicting the level of the mental well-being of the workers ($b = 0.02$; $p < 0.001$).

The workers who performed the greatest deep acting were found, in conditions of frequent, hostile customer behaviors, to be characterized by the poorest mental well-being.

3.11.1.3 Summary

In the private insurance employee group, the regression analysis revealed two interactive effects. Both concerned the role of deep acting in the relationship between hostile customer behaviors and the (physical and mental) well-being of workers. The high level of emotional labor was not detrimental to the well-being of workers in conditions of rare hostile customer behaviors. However, in conditions of frequent hostile customer behaviors, the poorest physical and mental well-being was experienced by those workers who did the highest levels of the deep acting.

3.11.2 SOCIAL INSURANCE WORKERS

3.11.2.1 The Moderating Role of Deep Acting in the Relationship between the Intensity of Hostile Customer Behaviors and the Physical Well-Being of Workers

An interactive component regression analysis showed that the deep acting–abusive customer behavior interaction effect was significant in predicting the level of the physical well-being of workers ($b = 0.02$; $p < 0.05$).

Those workers who did the highest levels of deep acting were found, in conditions of frequent hostile customer behaviors, to be characterized by the greatest physical well-being. In turn, the poorest physical well-being was observed among those workers who did the poorest level of deep acting in conditions of frequent, hostile customer behaviors.

3.11.2.2 The Moderating Role of Deep Acting in the Relationship between the Intensity of Hostile Customer Behaviors and the Mental Well-Being of Workers

The deep acting–hostile customer behaviors interaction effect was significant in predicting the level of the mental well-being of workers ($b = 0.01$; $p < 0.05$).

The greatest mental well-being was recorded among those workers who did most frequently the deep acting in conditions of frequent, hostile customer behaviors. In turn, those workers who did the lowest levels of emotional labor in conditions of frequent hostile customer behaviors were characterized by the poorest mental well-being.

3.11.2.3 The Moderating Role of Deep Acting in the Relationship between Disproportionate Customer Expectations and the Physical Well-Being of Workers

An interactive component regression analysis showed that the deep acting–disproportionate customer expectations interaction effect was significant in predicting the level of the physical well-being of employees ($b = 0.03$; $p < 0.05$).

The greatest physical well-being was observed among workers who did the greatest deep acting in conditions of frequent, disproportionate customer expectations. In turn, the poorest physical well-being was observed among those workers who, in conditions of frequent disproportionate customer expectations, did the lowest levels of deep acting.

3.11.2.4 The Moderating Role of Deep Acting in the Relationship between the Intensity of Disproportionate Customer Expectations and the Mental Well-Being of Workers

An interactive component regression analysis showed that the deep acting–disproportionate customer expectations interaction effect was significant in predicting the level of the mental well-being of workers ($b = 0.02$; $p < 0.05$).

The employees who used most frequently the deep acting strategy in conditions of frequent disproportionate customer expectations experienced the greatest mental well-being. In turn, the poorest mental well-being was observed among workers who, in conditions of frequent, disproportionate customer expectations performed the lowest levels of the deep acting.

3.11.2.5 The Moderating Role of Deep Acting in the Relationship between the Intensity of Disproportionate Customer Expectations and the Exhaustion of Employees

An interactive component regression analysis showed that the deep acting–disproportionate customer expectations interaction effect was significant in predicting the level of exhaustion of workers ($b = 0.03$; $p < 0.01$).

The lowest levels of exhaustion were observed among those employees who did the greatest levels of deep acting in conditions of frequent, disproportionate customer expectations. The most exhausted workers were found to be persons who, in conditions of frequent, disproportionate customer expectations recorded the poorest level of deep acting.

3.11.2.6 The Moderating Role of Faking Emotions in the Relationship between the Intensity of Disproportionate Customer Expectations and the Exhaustion of Employees

An interactive component regression analysis showed that the effect of the faking emotions–disproportionate customer expectations interaction was significant in predicting the level of employee exhaustion ($b = 0.02$; $p < 0.05$).

Those workers who most frequently faked emotions when interacting with customers in conditions of rare disproportionate customer expectations experienced the lowest levels of exhaustion. The most exhausted were those who, in conditions of rare disproportionate customer expectations, were the least likely to fake emotions. As the frequency of disproportionate customer expectations increased, employee exhaustion was exacerbated, regardless of the frequency of faking emotions, i.e. surface acting.

3.11.2.7 Summary

Six significant interactive effects have been observed in the group of social insurance workers. Five have been associated with deep acting. When confronted with frequent, hostile customer behaviors, workers who did the highest levels of deep acting experienced greater well-being (physical and mental) than workers with low levels of deep acting. In disproportionate customer expectations conditions, the best physical and mental well-being, as well as the lowest levels of exhaustion, were also observed among those workers who most frequently used the deep acting strategy. Conversely, the highest exhaustion was experienced by those workers who most frequently faked emotions when interacting with customers; however, this was the case only in rare disproportionate customer expectations conditions.

3.12 THE STUDY VARIABLES AND SICKNESS ABSENCE CORRELATION ANALYSIS

The analysis of the study results has been based on selected indicators of subjective questionnaire-based assessment of psychosocial working conditions, worker well-being, and customer relations. The well-being of workers has correlated with sickness absenteeism, which is an objective indicator of both worker health and well-being. In order to investigate which of the study variables are related to worker sickness absence, a correlational analysis of all study variables with the number of sick leave days in the preceding year has been conducted. The correlation analysis results of both study groups are presented in Table 3.7.

The correlation analysis results have confirmed the diversity of worker health and well-being factors in the employee study groups. In the private insurance employee group, sickness absence was found negatively correlated with disproportionate customer expectations ($r = -0.16$; $p < 0.05$), general well-being index ($r = -0.18$; $p < 0.05$), and the physical well-being of workers ($r = -0.19$; $p < 0.01$). The negative relationship between well-being and sickness absence seems to be straightforward. It is much more complex to depict the negative relationship between disproportionate customer expectations and sickness absence. The high intensity of disproportionate customer expectations has been associated with low sickness absence. It thus seems that private insurance workers may not be able to take days off due to illness during peak customer-demands periods.

Among the social insurance workers surveyed, sickness absence was negatively correlated with general well-being ($r = -0.16$; $p < 0.05$) and physical well-being ($r = -0.16$; $p < 0.05$), as in the case of private insurance workers. Moreover, statistically significant correlations with the cognitive control ($r = -0.14$; $p < 0.05$) and the emotional exhaustion ($r = 0.20$; $p < 0.01$) – a job burnout subscale – were observed. Social insurance workers who had clearly defined work objectives, job descriptions, working methods, access to information, and job security were less likely to be on sick leave. On the other hand, employees who were more emotionally exhausted were more likely to be off sick.

3.13 CONCLUSIONS

The statistical analysis has been carried out independently in two customer service employee groups and the following factors have been studied: sources of occupational stress and its consequences on the physical and mental health of workers, and intergroup differences in terms of tasks performed. The results have revealed

TABLE 3.7
Correlation Matrix between Study Variables and Sickness Absence in the Study Groups

		Disengagement from work	Exhaustion	Deep acting	Hiding feelings	Faking emotions	Abusive customer behavior	Disproportionate customer expectations	Job demands	Job control	Social support	Well-being	Expected changes	Intellectual demands	Psychophysical demands and responsibilities	Role conflict and workload demands	Behavioral control	Cognitive Control	Management social support	Co-worker social support	Physical well-being	Mental well-being
Sick leave absence																						
private insurance	r	-0.002	0.092	0.054	0.118	0.018	-0.003	-0.16*	-0.062	-0.104	-0.01	-0.18*	0.044	-0.061	0.007	-0.05	-0.136	-0.015	0.052	-0.072	-0.19**	-0.129
	p	0.977	0.198	0.447	0.099	0.802	0.967	0.028	0.387	0.145	0.894	0.013	0.538	0.395	0.917	0.488	0.057	0.836	0.469	0.316	0.008	0.071
social insurance	r	0.137	0.20**	-0.011	0.015	-0.059	0.003	-0.022	0.022	-0.098	-0.072	-0.16*	0.127	-0.001	-0.02	0.08	-0.031	-0.014*	-0.083	-0.04	-0.16*	-0.131
	p	0.053	0.005	0.874	0.838	0.406	0.963	0.752	0.761	0.169	0.312	0.028	0.073	0.988	0.778	0.26	0.663	0.044	0.242	0.577	0.023	0.064

r – Pearson correlation coefficient; p – significance level; * significant correlation at the $p < 0.05$ level; ** significant correlation at the $p < 0.01$ level differences in both the sources of stress and its effects. Each study group has its own specificity of psychosocial working conditions, customer relations, demographic characteristics and the experienced symptoms of job burnout, and physical and mental well-being. The following paragraphs present a discussion on the most important characteristics and dependencies identified for each employee study group.

Private insurance workers have been characterized by a low job burnout rate and a fairly high level of well-being (physical and mental well-being). In this group, a lower level of hiding feelings has been noted. Also, the private insurance workers declared a lower intensity level of hostile customer behaviors and disproportionate customer expectations. Hence, it can be concluded that in customer service work, this group represents low-intensity occupational stress results, which are conducive to the well-being of the surveyed workers.

Regarding the psychosocial working conditions in the private insurance group, a lower level of social support (by managers and co-workers alike) has been observed, which is an adverse factor. This may be due to the dominant form of independent task performance. Nevertheless, the private insurance employees have been found to enjoy a higher level of behavioral control – the autonomy in time and task performance management.

The regression analyses investigating the relationship between psychosocial working conditions and well-being and job burnout among private insurance employees have revealed that cognitive control is the strongest determinant of employee well-being and job burnout in this study group, as well as the predictive factor of all well-being and burnout indicators. The clearer the responsibilities, performance evaluation criteria, and working methods, and the greater the job security, the better the employees' mental and physical well-being, as well as the higher their work engagement and the lesser their exhaustion. In addition, co-worker social support, if received, has been found to improve mental well-being.

Of the two types of stress-inducing customer behaviors, only abusive customer behavior has been strongly associated with employee well-being and job burnout. The experience of such behaviors has been found to significantly deteriorate well-being and increase burnout rates in the private insurance employee group.

Regarding the emotional labor indicators, only hiding feelings (surface acting) has been associated with poorer well-being and higher job burnout. Deep acting has been associated with greater work engagement among private insurance employees.

The regression analyses have also revealed two interactive effects. They concerned the role of deep acting in the relationship between hostile customer behaviors and well-being (physical and mental) identified in the private insurance study group. The high level of emotional labor was not detrimental to the well-being of employees in conditions of low-intensity hostile customer behaviors. However, in conditions of frequent hostile customer behaviors, the poorest physical and mental well-being was experienced by those employees who did the greatest levels of deep acting. It thus seems that emotional engagement in customer service work is beneficial, but not when handling abusive customers.

The needs assessment analysis has shown that the expected changes concern mainly workload management, interpersonal communication, and social support areas.

The correlation analysis of sickness absence and the study variables has shown that disproportionate customer expectations are negatively associated with sickness absence. Therefore, private insurance employees cannot afford to be on sick leave during high customer demands peaks.

Social insurance workers have been characterized by a higher intensity of hiding feelings and more frequent exposure to hostile customer behaviors and disproportionate customer expectations. In terms of psychosocial working conditions, greater behavioral control over work objectives, responsibilities, working methods, access to information and job security have been observed in this study group. Such positive psychosocial factors have been found to mitigate the negative consequences of difficult customer relationships. Similarly, the higher level of social support received from both managers and co-workers has additionally attenuated the work-related stress among the social insurance workers. A lower physical well-being score has been recorded in this study group. This may be due to the higher mean age (43.8 years) of the social insurance workers surveyed, comparing to the private insurance workers (37.4 years).

The job demands in terms of role conflict, work overload, and behavioral control have been identified as the most important factors determining the well-being and job burnout of social insurance workers. Co-worker support has been found important for physical well-being, and management support has been significant for the mental well-being and work engagement of the employees.

Of the stress-inducing customer behavior types, only the abusive customer behavior has had a significant and very strong negative impact on the physical and mental wellbeing of social insurance workers. Hostile customer behaviors have also been strongly associated with higher levels of burnout noted in this employee group.

Regarding emotional labor, only the hiding-feelings surface acting has been related to the poorer well-being and greater job burnout of social insurance workers. In turn, deep acting has been associated with higher work engagement, i.e. lesser job burnout.

Six significant interactive effects have been identified in the social insurance employee group. Five effects have been associated with deep acting. When faced with high-intensity abusive customer behavior, workers who did a higher level of deep acting enjoyed a greater physical and mental well-being than workers who rarely used the deep acting emotional strategy. In conditions of disproportionate customer expectations, the greatest physical and mental well-being, with lesser exhaustion, was present among those workers who performed deep acting. Conversely, the greatest exhaustion was experienced by those workers who frequently faked emotions in customer interactions. However, in conditions of high-intensity, disproportionate customer expectations, the exhaustion level was similar regardless of the type of emotional labor performed.

The expected changes related mainly to increased skill-development opportunities, time and work management, as well as the presence of technical and IT equipment supporting task performance.

In the social insurance study group, sickness absence has been negatively correlated with the general and physical well-being of workers. Moreover, statistically significant correlations have been found between cognitive control and emotional exhaustion, an indicator of job burnout. Finally, social insurance workers who felt clear about their work objectives, job descriptions, and working methods, and who had access to the required information and enjoyed job security, were less likely to take sick leave. Conversely, those workers who were more emotionally exhausted were also more likely to be off sick.

The study results reveal the specificity of psychosocial working conditions in the context of job burnout, taking into account customer behaviors and types of emotional labor. In two occupational groups with a similar field of work but of two different forms (public administration versus private companies), differences have been observed both in the work properties and the influence of mediating factors. Apart from the type of emotional labor, other individual characteristics can be taken into account such as self-efficacy, or a Type A behavior pattern, considered in previous research. In the studies investigating the types of emotional labor, a limitation may be the potential divergence of worker emotional engagement from their health status in a given period, or acceptance of organizational principles at work. It could be further discussed whether the lack of emotional work engagement can also be considered a form of counterproductive behavior.

REFERENCES

Allen, J. A., J. M. Diefendorff, and Y. Ma. 2014. DOI: 10.1007/s10869-013-9288-7.

Austin, E. J., T. C. P. Dore, and K. M. O'Donovan. 2008. Associations of personality and emotional intelligence with display rule perceptions and emotional labour. *Pers Individ Dif* 44(3):679–688. DOI: 10.1016/j.paid.2007.10.001.

Baka, Ł., and B. A. Basińska. 2016. Psychometryczne właściwości polskiej wersji oldenburskiego kwestionariusza wypalenia zawodowego (OLBI). *Med Pr* 67(1):29–41.

Brotheridge, C. M. 2006. The role of emotional intelligence and other individual difference variables in predicting emotional labor relative to situational demands. *Psicothema* 18(Suppl. S):139–44.

Brotheridge, C. M., and A. A. Grandey. 2002. Emotional labour and burnout: Comparing two perspectives of "people work". *J Vocat Behav* 60(1):17–39. DOI: 10.1006/jvbe.2001.1815.

Brotheridge, C. M., and R. T. Lee. 2002. Testing a conservation of resources model of the dynamics of emotional labor. *J Occup Health Psychol* 7(1):57–67. DOI: 10.1037/1076-8998.7.1.57.

Cieślak, R., and M. Widerszal-Bazyl. 2000. *Psychospołeczne warunki pracy. Podręcznik do kwestionariusza*. Warszawa: CIOP.

Demerouti, E., A. B. Bakker, F. Nachreiner, and W. B. Schaufeli. 2001. The job demands–resources model of burnout. *J Appl Psychol* 86(3):499–512. DOI: 10.1037/0021-9010.86.3.499.

Dormann, C., and D. M. Kaiser. 2002. Job conditions and customer satisfaction. *Eur J Work Organ Psychol* 11(3):257–283. DOI: 10.1080/13594320244000166.

Finogenow, M., M. Wróbel, and J. Mróz. 2015. Skala płytkiej i głębokiej pracy emocjonalnej (SPGPE) – adaptacja narzędzia i analiza własności psychometrycznych. [Deep Acting and Surface Acting Scale (DASAS) – Adaptation of the method and preliminary psychometric properties]. *Med Pr* 66(3):359–371. DOI: 10.13075/mp.5893.00168.

Gopalan, N., S. S. Culbertson, and P. I. Leiva. 2012. Explaining emotional labor's relationship with emotional exhaustion and life satisfaction: Moderating role of perceived autonomy. *Univ Psychol* 12(2):347–356. DOI: 10.11144/Javeriana.UPSY12-2.eelr.

Grandey, A. A., G. M. Fisk, A. S. Mattila, K. J. Jansen, and L. A. Sideman. 2005. Is "service with a smile" enough? Authenticity of positive displays during service encounters. *Organ Behav Hum Decis Process* 96(1):38–55. DOI: 10.1016/j.obhdp.2004.08.002.

GUS [Główny Urząd Statystyczny]. 2014. Central Statistical Office, accidents at work and work-related health problems. https://stat.gov.pl/download/gfx/portalinformacyjny/pl/defaultaktualnosci/5476/2/2/7/pw:wypadki_przy_pracy_i_problemy_zdrow:zwiazane_z_praca.pdf (accessed January 23, 2020).

Hayes, A. F. 2013. *Introduction to Mediation, Moderation, and Conditional Process Analysis: A Regression-Based Approach.* New York: Guilford Press.

Hennig-Thurau, T., M. Groth, M. Paul, and D. Gremler. 2006. Are all smiles created equal? How emotional contagion and emotional labor affect service relationships. *J Mark* 70(3):58–73. DOI: 10.1509/jmkg.70.3.58.

Hochschild, A. 1983. *The Managed Heart: Commercialization of Human Feeling.* Berkeley, CA: University of California Press.

Jawahar, I. M., T. H. Stone, and J. L. Kisamore. 2007. Role conflict and burnout: The direct and moderating effects of political skill and perceived organizational support on burnout dimensions. *Int J Stress Manage* 14(2):142–159. DOI: 10.1037/1072-5245.14.2.142.

Jeung, D. Y., C. Kim, and S. J. Chang. 2018. Emotional labor and burnout: A review of the literature. *Yonsei Med J* 59(2):187–193. DOI: 10.3349/ymj.2018.59.2.187.

Karasek, R. A., and T. Theorell. 1990. *Healthy Work: Stress, Productivity and the Re-construction of Working Life.* New York: Basic Books.

Maneotis, S. M., A. A. Grandey, and A. D. Krauss. 2014. Understanding the "Why" as well as the "How": Service performance is a function of prosocial motives and emotional labor. *Hum Perform* 27(1):80–97. DOI: 10.1080/10503300802448899.

Maslach, C., and M. P. Leiter. 2008. Early predictors of job burnout and engagement. *J Appl Psychol* 93(3):498–512. DOI: 10.1037/0021-9010.93.3.498.

Maslach, C., W. B. Schaufeli, and M. P. Leiter. 2001. Job burnout. *Annu Rev Psychol* 52:397–422. DOI: 10.1146/annurev.psych.52.1.397.

Milczarek, M., and E. Brun. 2007. *Expert Forecast on Emerging Psychosocial Risks Related to Occupational Safety and Health.* Bilbao: European Agency for Safety and Health at Work.

Milczarek, M., E. Schneider, and E. R. Gonzales. 2009. *OSH in Figures: Stress at Work: Facts and Figures.* Bilbao: European Agency for Safety and Health at Work. https://osha.europa.eu/en/publications/osh-figures-stress-work-facts-and-figures (accessed January 23, 2020).

O'Connor, B. P. 1998. All-in-one programs for exploring interactions in moderated multiple regression. *Educ Psychol Meas* 58(5):833–837. DOI: 10.1177/0013164498058005009.

Ostrowska, M., and A. Michcik. 2013. Wypalenie zawodowe: Przyczyny, objawy, skutki, zapobieganie. *Bezpieczeństwo Pracy – Nauka i Praktyka* 8:22–25.

Sliter, M., Y. Chen, S. Withrow, and K. Sliter. 2013. Older and (emotionally) smarter? Emotional intelligence as a mediator in the relationship between age and emotional labor strategies in service employees. *Exp Aging Res* 39(4):466–479. DOI: 10.1080/0361073X.2013.808105.

Szczygieł, D., and R. Bazińska. 2013. Emotional intelligence as a moderator in the relationship between negative emotions and emotional exhaustion among employees in service sector occupations. *Polish Psychol Bull* 44(2):201–212. DOI: 10.2478/ppb-2013-0023.

Szczygieł, D., R. Bazinska, R. Kadzikowska-Wrzosek, and S. Retowski. 2009. Praca emocjonalna w zawodach usługowych: Pojęcie, przegląd teorii i badań. *Psychol Społeczna* 4(11):155–166.

Wróbel, M. 2013. Praca emocjonalna a wypalenie zawodowe u nauczycieli: Moderująca rola inteligencji emocjonalnej. *Psychol Społeczna* 8(24):53–66.

4 Health Impairment Process in Human Service Work

The Role of Emotional Demands and Personal Resources

Łukasz Baka

CONTENTS

The study group were youth rehabilitation center workers ($N = 200$). The study sample selection criteria were for the special character profession involving intensive and direct contact with other people, coupled with the provision of assistance job demand. The measurement tools were the Copenhagen Psychosocial Questionnaire (COPSOQ II), the Oldenburg Burnout Inventory (OLBI), and the Center for Epidemiologic Studies Depression Scale (CES-D).

The study results have largely confirmed the job demands–resources model. Emotional job demands were not directly related to depression but led to it indirectly through increased job burnout. The buffering role of personal resources has only partially been supported by the empirical evidence. Among the tested moderation effects, only the relation between the hiding emotions job demand and job burn-out was confirmed. The obtained results, apart from cognitive values, offer useful information for psychological practice. The results show that strengthening indi-vidual worker resources can be part of prevention programs, including coping with stress and reducing the risk of burnout among persons employed in social mission occupations.

4.1   INTRODUCTION

According to a recently published WHO report, depression is the second leading cause of disability worldwide [Ferrari et al. 2013]. Studies show that approximately 7% of European citizens suffer from depression annually [Wittchen et al. 2010]; however, over 41% of the European population experience at least one episode of depression during their lifetime [Moffitt, Caspi, and Taylor 2010]. Depression is also cited as one of the main causes of work incapacity, or a poor work ability [Steadman and Taskila 2015; Whiteford et al. 2013]. The costs of depression affect workers, employers, and society as a whole. In Poland, mental disorders are the third cause of the longest periods of absence from work after cancer and pregnancy, and account for almost 8% of all sick-leave days per year In 2017, the mental-disorders-related sick-leave absence amounted to over 10 million calendar days [Żołnierczyk-Zreda and Holas 2018].

Apart from hereditary conditions, environmental factors [Butcher, Hooley, and Mineka 2018], including psychosocial hazards at the workplace [e.g. Theorell et al. 2015] are underlined in the etiology of depression. Meta-analyses of studies con-ducted in recent years indicate the important role of the work environment in the development of depression [Bonde 2008; Madsen et al. 2017; Netterstrøm et al. 2008; Niedhammer, Malard, and Chastang 2015; Nieuwenhuijsen, Bruinvels, and Frings-Dresen 2010; Rugulies and Madsen 2017], but the mechanisms for its development and methods of reducing the risk of its occurrence remain unclear.

A more recent occupational stress model, the Job Demand–Resources (JD–R) model [Bakker and Demerouti 2017; Schaufeli and Bakker 2004] has been an attempt to explain these dynamics by referring to the mediating role of job burn-out. The authors of the model have identified dual processes that play a role in the development of job-related strain and motivation [Bakker and Demerouti 2007]. In the first process, coined the "motivational process", job resources lead to desirable organizational outcomes (e.g. organizational commitment) via work engagement. According to the second process, coined the "health impairment process", prolonged job demands result in diminished job resources, which is conducive to job burnout and leads to depression in the long run [Bakker and Demerouti 2007]. The health impairment process has been the focus of the current study. It has been supported by previous research findings [Baka 2015; de Beer, Pienaar, and Rothmann 2016; Hakanen, Bakker, and Schaufeli 2006; Hakanen, Schaufeli, and Ahola 2008; Hu, Schaufeli, and Taris 2011; Lewig et al. 2007], however, most of the studies have been conducted following the cross-sectional study paradigm, and not the cross-lagged study method. This has been problematic as testing mediation effects based on the results of cross-sectional studies is being heavily criticized in social research

[Maxwell, Cole, and Mitchell 2011]. Researchers have pointed out that the cross-sectional method, measuring study variables at a single point in time, does not permit the establishment of a clear causal relationship between variables. The classical mediation method developed by Baron and Kenny [1986] and the Sobel test [1982] have also been criticized, and more recent and effective research methods have been proposed as a result [Rucker et al. 2011; Williams and MacKinnon 2008].

Furthermore, most of the cited studies on the health impairment process have mainly focused on workload-related job demands (e.g. quantitative workload, work pace, time pressure), work content (e.g. task demands) and roles (role conflict, role ambiguity, unclear decision-making structures), omitting somewhat emotional job demands related to experiences of negative emotions at work, emotional control, or emotional labor. Emotional demands have now been identified as one of the most burdensome factors in the work environment, which is also due to the increase in the number and intensity of daily interpersonal contacts at work, including both direct human contact and modern technology communication processes. Relationships consisting in intensive and direct contact with other people, coupled with a job requirement to provide various forms of assistance, such as care for socially excluded or disadvantaged persons, or those in conflict with the law, are particularly emotionally demanding [Soderfeldt et al. 1996].

According to the JD–R model, high resources buffer the negative effects of job demands and reduce the risk of mental health problems [Bakker et al. 2003]. As far as the beneficial role of job resources (e.g. social support, job control) has been widely supported by empirical studies [Bakker et al. 2003; Bakker, Demerouti, and Euwema 2005], the research has produced inconsistent results on the role of personal resources [e.g. Heuven et al. 2006; Xanthopolou, Bakker, and Schaufeli 2007]. The aim of the one-year cross-lagged study presented in the current chapter is to investigate the mechanism of depression incidence in a group of youth rehabilitation center and youth hostel employees. A particular focus has been placed on examining the direct and indirect effects (mediated by job burnout) of emotional demands on depression and on investigating moderational effects of personal resources on direct and indirect effects of emotional demands.

4.2 EMOTIONAL DEMANDS IN HUMAN SERVICE WORK

The Job Demands–Control (JDC) model [Karasek 1979; Karasek and Theorell 1990], developed in the late 1970s and considered the most robust occupational stress model, points to the interaction of high job demands and low job control as the main cause of health problems at work. Karasek's job demands were mainly quantitative demands, e.g. the amount of work, work pace, time pressure. The emphasis on this type of job demands mainly stems from the industrial work environment analysis that the model was built on. In the critique of the JDC model, Söderfeldt et al. have reproached the neglect of the burdensome role of emotional demands [Soderfeldt et al. 1996], which are crucial for employees of human service organizations whose "principal function is to protect, maintain, or enhance the personal well-being of individuals by defining, shaping, or altering their personal attributes" [Hasenfeld 1974]. Soderfeldt et al. [1996] have suggested that workers in human service organizations face specific, albeit different than industrial, types of job demands that require close emotional relationships with other people and active involvement in their problems. As the authors write: "There are also special emotional demands, due to the nature of the work. Workers in human service organizations are confronted with poverty, disease, criminality and many other facets of human problems and suffering, together with gnawing feelings of own inadequacy" [Soderfeldt et al. 1996]. The authors of the JD–R model have depicted job demands more broadly as physical, psychological, social, or organizational aspects of the job that require sustained physical and/ or psychological effort [Bakker and Demerouti 2017] and have considered emotional demands at work as a source of job strain.

Emotional demands are defined as "those aspects of the job that require sustained emotional effort" [Zapf 2002]. In human service work, they usually concern two kinds of situations. The first type is related to emotionally burdensome relations with other people (e.g. long-term care, interpersonal conflicts, supervision of aggressive people) and the amount and intensity of negative emotional experiences (e.g. anxiety, anger, hostility, sadness) in the workplace. The consequences of negative emotional experiences are an increase in stress levels [Moskowitz, 2001; Mayne 2001], followed by a deterioration in mental and physical health [Gross 1989; Kemeny and Shestyuk 2008; Consedine 2008]. The second type concerns the requirement to observe the emotional *display rules* [cf. Ekman 1973] in interpersonal contacts (e.g. with a co-worker, supervisor, patient, pupil), consisting in showing positive emotions and hiding negative ones [Beal et al. 2006; Hochschild 1983]. The act of emotional regulation according to the set organizational standards has been associated with negative health consequences [Hochschild 1983; Brotheridge and Grandey 2002; Van Maanen and Kunda 1989]. Researchers have argued that emotional regulation at work, just like any other form of self-regulation, requires effort and therefore depletes the personal resources of the employee, which may result in poorer health [cf. Gross 1989]. In the present research, both types of emotional demands have been taken into account.

Several prospective studies on human service organization employees have confirmed the positive relationship between emotional demands and job burnout [Sundin et al. 2007; Idris, Dollard, and Yulita 2014; Lorente Prieto et al. 2008; van Vegchel et al. 2004], and depression [Andrea et al. 2009; Kim, Noh, and Muntaner 2013; Muntaner et al. 2006]. A one-year interval measurement study conducted by van Vegchel et al. [2004] revealed an association between emotional demands (e.g. handling troublesome clients) and emotional exhaustion among social insurance employees. Similar results were obtained by Lorente Prieto et al. [2008] in an eight-month interval measurement study carried out in a group of 274 schoolteachers. Regarding the research on depression, high emotional demands (e.g. unfair treatment, patient's family abuse, unmet care needs, patient health, and emotional suppression) predicted the incidence of depression measured after 6 months in a group of 1,599 home care workers [Kim et al. 2013], and measured after 2 years in a group of nursing assistance workers [Muntaner et al. 2006]. In two prospective studies, emotional demands at baseline predicted the subsequent use of antidepressants [Madsen, Diderichsen, and Rugulies 2010; Magnusson Hanson et al. 2013], and were also associated with hospitalization for clinical depression in a case-control study based on a job-exposure matrix of work-related psychosocial exposures, although only for women [Wieclaw et al. 2008].

4.3 DIRECT EFFECT OF JOB DEMANDS ON DEPRESSION

Depression is an affective disorder characterized by depressed mood, loss of interest or pleasure, and decreased energy accompanied by symptoms such as feelings of guilt or low self-esteem, disturbed sleep or appetite, and poor concentration [Butcher, Hooley, and Mineka 2018]. In addition to the relationship between depression and emotional demands described in the previous paragraph, researchers have also pointed to the role of other psychosocial working conditions in the development of depression. The results of studies on the direct relationship between psychosocial risks at work and depression have been inconsistent. A significant part of cross-sectional studies shows positive dependencies [Baka 2015; Chen et al. 2009; Siegrist 2008], however, meta-analysis study results [Bonde 2008; Madsen et al. 2017; Netterstrøm et al. 2008; Nieuwenhuijsen, Bruinvels, and Frings-Dresen 2010; Rugulies and Madsen 2017; Theorell et al. 2015] have been less coherent. Particularly noteworthy are the prospective studies conducted with an interval between the initial and final measurement of not less than one year on large study samples [Netterstrøm et al. 2008; Theorell et al. 2015; Żołnierczyk-Zreda and Holas 2018]. These include national projects involving many study participant cohorts, such as the *Netherlands Mental Health Survey and Incidence Study* (NEMESIS), the *Maastricht Cohort Study on Fatigue at Work*, the Belgian *Job Stress Project* (BELSTRESS), the British *Whitehall II*, the Danish *Psychosocial Risk Factors for Stress and Mental Disease* study (PRISME), the French *Santé et Itinéraire Professionnel* (SIP), or the *Canadian National Population Health Survey*. In those studies, depression was diagnosed based on both subjective assessment of the respondents and the opinion of a specialized clinician.

Accordingly, the NEMESIS project examined 2,646 workers twice, with a two-year interval between measurements, for different types of psychosocial risks. The results showed that high psychological demands (but not job insecurity, nor low job control) predicted the incidence of depression after two years since the first measurement [Plaisier et al. 2007]. Similar results were obtained in the BELSTRESS project in a group of 2,821 employees, conducted with a measurement interval of over 6.5 years [Clays et al. 2007]. In the French SIP project, Niedhammer, Malard, and Chastang [2015] examined 4,717 employees twice – with a four-year interval – for job demands (i.e. quantitative workload, emotional demands, role conflict, job insecurity, ethical conflict, effort-reward imbalance and work–life imbalance), job resources (job control and social support) and depression. The study results revealed that only high job insecurity and high effort–reward imbalance were associated with depression measured four years after the first measurement. The Canadian study used nationwide population health data on over 20,000 people and demonstrated that *day-to-day stress* and low social support were associated with depression, measured after one year since the first measurement [Shields 2006].

4.4   MEDIATION EFFECT OF JOB BURNOUT IN
JOB DEMANDS – DEPRESSION LINK

In order to investigate the inconsistencies identified in study findings on the associations between job demands and depression, the authors of the J–DR model have referred to the role of job burnout as a mediating variable in the job demands–depression relationship [Bakker and Demerouti 2007; Bakker and Demerouti 2017]. Job burnout, which is a long-term effect of chronic work-related stress caused by excessive job demands, constitutes a potential mediator derived from the work-related domain. In the present study, a two-dimensional definition of job burnout has been applied [Demerouti et al. 2001], suggesting that job burnout consists of exhaustion and disengagement from work. Exhaustion is a response to intensive physical, affective, and cognitive strain. It is manifested in fatigue, weariness, and a decrease in vitality. Disengagement from work is expressed by distancing oneself from work and by experiencing negative work-related affect [Demerouti et al. 2001].

According to the JD–R model, depression develops over time and is a postponed response to stressful environmental factors. As reported by the model's authors, job demands first lead to a "depletion" of resources associated with stress management, which over time results in exhaustion and reduced work engagement. A prolonged depletion and lack of resources are conducive to depression over time. Explaining the mediation effect of job burnout, Bakker and Demerouti [2007] have referred to the *compensatory regulatory-control model* [Hockey 1997]. According to the model, protracted job demands result in the mobilization of employee effort in order to maintain the required level of performance. However, this is associated with high psychophysiological costs – activation of the sympathetic system, irritability, or fatigue. A sustained high level of stressors gradually depletes the employee's resources needed to cope with stress (e.g. time, energy, mental and physical strength, abilities, equipment, social support). This can lead to professional burnout and, as a result, to poorer mental health. Indeed, meta-analysis studies have shown that the strongest determinant of job burnout is the high level of chronic job demands [Lee and Ashforth 1996], whereas a prolonged job burnout is a strong determinant of ill-health symptoms [Melamed et al. 2006]. Numerous cross-sectional studies [e.g. Bakker et al 2003; Hakanen, Bakker, and Schaufeli 2006; Lewig et al. 2007; Rothmann and Essenko 2007; Schaufeli and Bakker 2004] and several cross-lagged studies [Hakanen, Schaufeli, and Ahola 2008; de Beer, Pienaar, and Rothmann 2016] have confirmed the mediating mechanism of job burnout in the health impairment process within the JD–R framework.

4.5   MODERATION EFFECT OF PERSONAL RESOURCES

The JD–R model initially focused on the role of job resources as a stress buffer [Demerouti et al. 2001]. Research has confirmed that various types of job resources (e.g. social support, job control, psychological climate, feedback, coaching) facilitate coping with high job demands [Schaufeli and Bakker 2004]. Over time, the authors of the JD–R model have expanded the tool on personal resources as a significant factor in coping with job demands. Personal resources constitute cognitive and effective personality traits subject to a learning process and framed as positive beliefs about oneself (self-esteem, optimism, self-efficacy) and the social environment (optimism, hope), which motivate to achieve one's own goals, even in the face of adverse conditions and high expectations [van den Heuvel, Demerouti, and Schaufeli 2010]. Personal resources concern an individual perception of the ability to control the environment successfully [Hobfoll 1989]. Their main functions are to enable the individual to effectively handle difficult situations perceived as a challenge, and to facilitate the achievement of objectives [van den Heuvel, Demerouti, and Schaufeli 2010].

Research on the beneficial role of personal resources has produced inconsistent results so far [Heuven et al. 2006; Jex and Bliese 1999; Szczygieł and Baka 2016; Xanthopolou, Bakker, and Schaufeli 2007]. For example, in a study conducted among airplane cabin crew attendants, Heuven et al. [2006] proved that self-efficacy reduced the negative impact of emotional demands on exhaustion. In other studies, organizational-based self-esteem [Jex and Bliese 1999], self-efficacy [Van Yperen and Snijders 2000], optimism [Mäkikangas and Kinnunen 2003], emotional intelligence [Szczygieł and Baka 2016], and compassion satisfaction [Tremblay and Messervey 2011] moderated the effect of job demands on mental health. However, the moderating effect of personal resources (e.g. self-efficacy, self-esteem, and optimism) was not confirmed on a large sample of 1,121 Dutch employees [Xanthopolou, Bakker, and Schaufeli 2007].

These studies have accounted for self-efficacy, defined as generalized beliefs about the possibility of effective action in new, ambiguous or unpredictable situations [Bandura 1997]. This construct is not treated by Bandura as an individual-differences or personality-traits variable. Self-efficacy refers to the representation of a latent knowledge about oneself, more specifically, the knowledge on the effects of personal actions in situations important for the *self*. Thus, it co-determines individual thoughts and emotions in stressful conditions, and impacts upon motivation in undertaking actions to achieve the goal. A significant part of human activity and actions, before they are implemented, is carried out in the mind of the individual. Bandura [1997] claims that self-efficacy beliefs determine individually created scenarios. Persons characterized by a strong self-confidence in unexpected or important life circumstances create more optimistic scenarios and opportunities, and fewer risks, comparing to persons with low self-efficacy levels. Consequently, the latter establish more ambitious targets and are more committed to achieving them. The association between aspirations and the sense of effectiveness is a mutual relationship – the achievement of a challenging goal reinforces the sense of self-efficacy, which has a positive impact on the setting of ever more ambitious goals, and even yields an active search for challenging opportunities.

The following four research hypotheses have been put forward in relation to the direct effect of job demands on depression, the indirect effect of job burnout, and the moderation effect of self-efficacy.

H1: Emotional demands at work are positively associated with depression
H2: Job burnout mediates the negative effects of emotional demands at work
    on depression

H3: Self-efficacy buffers the negative effects of emotional demands at work
   on job burnout

H4: Self-efficacy buffers the negative effects of emotional demands at work
   on depression

4.6 METHOD

4.6.1 PARTICIPANTS AND PROCEDURE

The surveyed persons ($N = 200$) were employees of social rehabilitation centers –
youth education centers, youth sociotherapy centers, youth hostels, and correctional
facilities. In terms of numbers, women prevailed: $n = 156$ (78%), and the men num-
bered $n = 44$ (22%). The age of the respondents was between 24 and 70 years, and the
average age was 43.2 (SD = 9.27). Most respondents had completed higher education
(87.5%) or secondary education (8.5%). The average career length in the occupation
was 14.1 years (SD = 9.85).

A cross-lagged, one-year measurement interval study was conducted in the period
from September to November 2017 and 2018 by trained research assistants at the
study participants' employment premises. All participants were treated in compliance with the ethical guidelines of the Declaration of Helsinki. Participants received
a hard copy of the questionnaires along with a letter explaining the purpose of the
study. Full data confidentiality and anonymity were ensured. Participants were asked
to fill out the questionnaires and seal them in envelopes, which were subsequently
collected by the research assistants. Out of 500 distributed questionnaires, 358 (72%)
were returned and 200 (40% of the original pool) were at least 75% complete and
subsequently used for data analysis.

4.6.1.1 Measure

Emotional demands at work were measured with two COPSOQ II subscales
[Pejtersen, Kristensen, and Borg 2010] related to the frequency of burdensome interpersonal relationships (four-item emotional demands subscale) and hiding emotions
demands (three-item hiding emotions demands subscale). Both subscales had a five-
point answer scale, with responses from 1 (Always) to 5 (Never/Hardly ever).

Personal resources were measured with the COPSOQ II self-efficacy subscale,
comprising 6 items, with answers ranging from 1 *(Fits perfectly)* to 4 *(Does not fit)*.

Job burnout was measured with the Oldenburg Burnout Inventory [Demerouti
et al. 2001]. This 16-item scale comprises two subscales corresponding to exhaustion
and disengagement from work. The global index of burnout has been applied in the
present study. A 5-point response scale ranged from 1 *(I completely disagree)* to 5
(I completely agree).

Depression was measured with the CES-D instrument [Radloff 1977]. This scale
comprises 20 statements that measure the frequency of depressive symptoms experienced in the past week. The statements relate to depressed mood, feelings of guilt
and hopelessness, psychomotor slowdown, and sleep disorders. A 4-point answer
scale ranged from 0 – *rarely*, or *not at all (less than one day)* to 3 – *most of the time*
or *all the time (5–7 days)*.

4.6.1.2 Analytical Procedure

Prior to the main analyses, descriptive statistics were calculated, and correlation analysis was carried out. To verify the hypotheses, the structural equations modeling (SEM) method from AMOS statistical software was used. It is a method based on regression equations that allows testing research hypotheses with a high possibility of complex relationships between variables. The model tested: (1) direct effect of emotional demands at work on depression; (2) indirect effect of job burnout on the emotional demands at work – depression link; (3) the interactional effects of emotional demands at work and personal resources on job burnout and depression. The following factors were introduced to the model: emotional demands (T1), hiding emotions demands (T1), personal resources (T1), job burnout (T2) and depression (T2). Prior to the main study analyses, descriptive statistics were calculated, and correlation analysis and confirmatory factor analysis (CFA) of the tools used in the structure proposed by its authors were carried out to determine the factor accuracy and estimate the fitting parameters. The following data fit measures were used: *Root Mean Square Error of Approximation* (RMSEA), *Standardized Root Mean Squared Residual* (SRMR), *Comparative Fit Index* (CFI) and *Tucker–Lewis Index* (TLI). Despite the lack of a unanimous agreement, some authors suggest that values of CFI and TLI > 0.90, RMSEA < 0.05 and SMRM < 0.08 show a good data fit of the model. However, the accepted values are CFI and TLI > 0.85, RMSEA < 0.08 and SMRM < 0.10 [Byrne 2010; Kline 2011; Sharma 1996]. The analysis of the internal consistency of the study tools was also conducted using the Omega coefficient, which is more adequate in the analysis of latent factors than the Alpha coefficient. The Alpha coefficients were provided for reference as they are the more frequently used values in statistical analysis.

4.6.1.3 Results

Table 4.1 presents the correlation analysis results. It shows that gender is positively associated with self-efficacy and negatively associated with emotional demands. The Student's t-test analysis showed significant differences in this respect: women were characterized by lower self-efficacy and higher emotional demands than men. The results have also revealed that career length is positively correlated with emotional demands – the greater the career length, the higher the level of emotional demands. Age has not been associated with the independent, nor mediating or dependent, variables analyzed. Regarding the direct relationship between two types of emotional job demands and job burnout, and depression, hiding emotions demands (T1) have been associated both with job burnout (T2) and, slightly less, with depression (T2), while emotional demands (T1) have positively correlated only with professional burnout (T2). Self-efficacy (T1) has not been directly related to job burnout (T2) nor depression (T2) but has shown a positive association with emotional demands (T1). A strong relationship between job burnout (T2) and depression (T2) has also been identified.

Table 4.2 presents the CFA results showing the data fit parameters of the study tools. The results demonstrate that the tools used have satisfactory statistical parameters. The RMSEA measures are below the required threshold of 0.08, the SRMR measures below the threshold of 0.1, while the CFI and TLI values of most tools are above the 0.85 threshold. The reliability Cronbach's α and McDonalds' Ω coefficients fall above 0.75 value and are also satisfactory.

TABLE 4.1

The Correlation Analysis Results of the Analyzed Variables

	1	2	3	4	5	6	7	8	M	SD
Age (T1)	—									
Gender (T1)	-0.12*	—								
Career length (T1)	0.68***	-0.08	—							
Emotional demands (T1)	0.05	-0.13*	0.13*	—						
Hiding emotions demands (T1)	0.01	-0.06	0.05	0.31***	—					
Self-efficacy (T1)	-0.06	0.11*	-0.01	0.15**	0.02	—				
Job burnout (T2)	-0.03	-0.03	0.01	0.20**	0.24***	-0.06	—			
Depression (T2)	0.02	-0.04	0.08	0.01	0.11*	-0.05	0.39***	—		

$*p < 0.05$; $**p < 0.01$; $***p < 0.001$

TABLE 4.2

Data Fit Parameters of the Study Tools and Reliability Factors

	RMSEA	CFI	TLI	SRMR	Omega	α
Emotional demands	0.060	0.988	0.977	0.062	0.798	0.804
Hiding emotions demands	0.068	0.849	0.841	0.089	0.704	0.839
Self-efficacy	0.030	0.906	0.858	0.048	0.819	0.874
Job burnout	0.071	0.878	0.866	0.093	0.834	0.891
Depression	0.063	0.871	0.804	0.086	0.882	0.843

Note: RMSEA – Root Mean Square Error of Approximation; SRMR – standardized root mean squared residual; CFI – Comparative Fit Index; TLI – Tucker–Lewis Index.

The structural equations analysis has only partially confirmed the research hypotheses (Figure 4.1). It has proved that there is no association between depression (T2) and the two indicators of emotional demands at work (T1): emotional demands ($\beta = -0.017$; ns) and hiding emotions demands ($\beta = 0.046$ ns). The predicted direct effect, in *H1*, of emotional demands at work on depression has not been confirmed either. Regarding the mediating role of job burnout, the statistical analysis has confirmed that job burnout (T2) fully mediates the emotional demands at work–depression (T1–T2) relationship. It has proven that both emotional demands ($\beta = 0.118$; $p < 0.05$) and hiding emotions demands ($\beta = 0.166$; $p < 0.01$) lead to an increase in job burnout, which in turn is strongly associated with depression ($\beta = 0.413$; $p < 0.001$). Thus, *H2* can be considered fully confirmed. Regarding the buffering role of personal resources, the analysis has shown that self-efficacy (T1) mitigates the negative effect of hiding emotions demands (but not emotional demands) on job burnout ($\beta = 0.110$; $p < 0.05$). Figure 4.2 shows the observed moderation effect

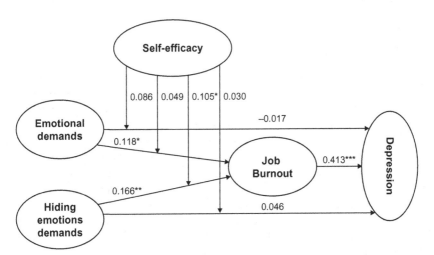

FIGURE 4.1 Direct effect of job demands, indirect effect of job burnout and moderation effect of personal resources on depression.

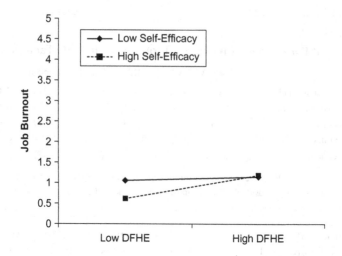

FIGURE 4.2 Moderational effect of personal resources on the hiding emotions demands–job burnout relationship.

of self-efficacy. Accordingly, employees with high self-efficacy are characterized by a lower level of job burnout, but only in conditions of low hiding emotions job demands. In conditions of high hiding emotions demands, there are no observed differences in terms of job burnout among persons with low and high self-efficacy. In other words, self-efficacy moderates the effect of job demands but only to a certain point. When hiding emotions demands grow, self-efficacy no longer has a beneficial effect. However, no moderating self-efficacy role has been observed in the emotional demands at work–depression relationship. Based on the obtained results, it can be concluded that *H3* has been partially confirmed, whereas *H4 has not* been confirmed.

4.7 DISCUSSION

The aim of the study was to determine the longitudinal impact of job demands on the development of depression in a group of youth rehabilitation center employees. Given the inconsistent previous research findings on the direct relationship between job demands and depression, both the direct effect of job demands, and the mediating role of other job-related variables, have been taken into account. The authors of the JD–R model indicate job burnout and the health-impairment process as key mediators in the impact of occupational stress on health [Bakker and Demerouti 2007]. The health-impairment process has been tested in the present study. Two types of job demands – emotional demands and hiding emotions demands – have been analyzed as core characteristics of various youth rehabilitation centers employees' work. The youth rehabilitation service work is classified as a human service profession, defined as a professional activity focused on providing assistance, satisfying the basic needs of other people, ensuring physical and health security, and providing people with basic skills or knowledge enabling them to function in society. Thus, human service professions should be mainly characterized by the motivation and the willingness to help and care for others – both their current and future well-being. This is often associated with a high level of responsibility for the people who are direct beneficiaries of the professional activity. In these professions, a close, engaging relationship with another person and emotional exchange processes constitute the foundation of the professional work. A teacher, educator or pedagogue her/himself is the basic "tool" of the educational and therapeutic process and its effectiveness.

The conducted cross-lagged study results have not supported the direct relationship between job demands and depression. The results have shown that both emotional demands and hiding emotions demands are not associated with depression measured after a one-year interval since the first measurement. However, the mediation effects analysis has proven that professional burnout plays a key role in the development of depression. High job demands measured in T1 led to an increase in the job burnout measured in T2, and this resulted in an increase in the depression measured in T2. The obtained results have supported the health-impairment process and have been consistent with the compensatory regulatory-control model [Hockey 1997]. The model upholds that working environment hazards affect the employee in a long-term manner and that their effects are deferred in time. In the first phase of coping with job demands, the employee mobilizes the strength, commitment, and effort needed to carry out professional tasks to maintain the required level of work quality and performance. This effort is accompanied by activation of the sympathetic system – e.g. increase in cortisol levels [Melamed et al. 1999] – and evokes somatic responses that disturb the anabolic and catabolic (metabolic) processes in the affected individuals [Ekstedt et al. 2006]. This gradually exhausts the employee's resources to cope with stress, resulting in job burnout and subsequent mental problems.

It is worth noting the identified distinction between challenge and hindrance stressors used in psychology [Cavanaugh et al. 2000]. Challenge stressors refer to those job demands perceived by the employee as creating opportunities for personal development – gaining new skills, experiences, broadening horizons, strengthening self-efficacy. Hence, they can be a source of positive emotions and have a motivating effect. In turn, hindrance-stressors are associated with job demands that conflict with other duties at work and impede the achievement of goals and personal development, and therefore have a more negative impact on the mental health of workers [Boswell, Olson-Buchanan, and LePine 2004]. In a study conducted by Bakker and Sanz-Vergel [2013], the researchers suggested that whether a given demand would be classified in a challenge or a hindrance group depended on the specificity of the work. As an example, the authors provided quantitative demands and emotional demands to human service work (e.g. nurses) and other occupational group professions (e.g. journalists). Tight deadlines are a daily problem for journalists because newspapers and news programs are usually distributed and broadcast daily. Hence, journalists consider time pressure as a challenge. In the case of nurses, time pressure is a hindrance because it means that there is not enough time to provide the patients with the care they need, which is conducive to professional fatigue and frustration. Conversely, emotional demands in nursing work (i.e. frequent interactions with patients and handling patient's emotions and family) represent "the heart of the work" [Bakker and Vergel 2013] and are considered a challenge. The present study results have not confirmed this premise. However, the results have shown that emotional demands at work are a source of job burnout in the studied group of human service work employees.

The beneficial role of personal resources (self-efficacy) has also been partially confirmed. They moderated the effect of hiding emotions demands (but not emotional demands) on professional burnout. These results are consistent with the JD–R model [Bakker and Demerouti 2017] and previous research findings [Heuven et al. 2006; Jex and Bliese 1999]. The present study, apart from cognitive values, also offers useful knowledge for the psychological practice. The study has revealed that strengthening self-efficacy may be an element of preventive programs covering stress management strategies and reducing the risk of burnout among rehabilitation center employees. This is particularly true since, as Bandura [1997] emphasizes, self-efficacy is to a large extent influenced by the environment, including the professional environment. Self-efficacy is built upon the opinions of important persons (e.g. managers), one's own experience (e.g. successes in projects), and an observed effectiveness of other persons' behavior (e.g. co-workers). Therefore, it is particularly important to provide employees with reliable feedback at task-performance level, to set realistic requirements that can be met by employees, and to enable them to learn from their leaders.

REFERENCES

Andrea, H., U. Bültmann, L. G. P. M. van Amelsvoort, and Y. Kant. 2009. The incidence of anxiety and depression among employees: The role of psychosocial work characteristics. *Depress Anxiety* 26(11):1040–1048.

Baka, Ł. 2015. Does job burnout mediate negative effects of job demands on mental and physical health in group of teachers? Testing the energetic process in job demands-resources model. *Int J Occup Med Environ Health* 28(2):335–346.

Bakker, A. B., and A. I. Sanz-Vergel. 2013. Weekly work engagement and flourishing: The role of hindrance and challenge demands. *J Vocat Behav* 83(3):397–409.

Bakker, A. B., and E. Demerouti. 2007. The job demands-resources model: State of the art. *J Managerial Psychol* 22(3):309–328.

Bakker, A. B., and E. Demerouti. 2017. Job demands-resources theory: Taking stock and looking forward. *J Occup Health Psychol* 22(3):273–285.

Bakker, A. B., E. Demerouti, E. De Boer, and W. Schaufeli. 2003. Job demands and job resources as predictors of absence duration and frequency. *J Vocat Behav* 62:341–356.

Bakker, A. B., E. Demerouti, and M. C. Euwema. 2005. Job resources buffer the impact of job demands on burnout. *J Occup Health Psychol* 10(2):170–180.

Bandura, A. 1997. *Self – efficacy: The exercise control.* New York: W.H. Freeman.

Baron, R. M., and Kenny, D. A. 1986. The moderator – mediator variable distinction in social psychological research. Conceptual, strategic and statistical considerations. *Pers Soc Psychol* 51(6):1173–1182.

Beal, D. J., J. P. Trougakos, H. M. Weiss, and S. G. Green. 2006. Episodic processes in emotional labor: Perceptions of affective delivery and regulation strategies. *J Appl Psychol* 91(5):1053–1065.

Bonde, J. P. E. 2008. Psychosocial factors at work and risk of depression: A systematic review of the epidemiological evidence. *Occup Environ Med* 65:438–445.

Boswell, W. R., J. B. Olson-Buchanan, and M. A. LePine. 2004. Relations between stress and work outcomes: The role of felt challenge, job control, and psychological strain. *J Vocat Behav* 64(1):165–181.

Brotheridge, C. M., and A. A. Grandey. 2002. Emotional labor and burnout: Comparing two perspectives of "people work". *J Vocat Behav* 760(1):17–39.

Butcher, J. N., J. M. Hooley, and S. Mineka. 2018. *Abnormal psychology. DSM-5*. New York: Pearson Editing.

Byrne, B. M. 2010. *Structural equation modeling with AMOS. Basic concepts, applications, and programming*. New York: Routledge/Taylor & Francis Group.

Cavanaugh, M. A., W. R. Boswell, M. V. Roehling, and J. W. Boudreau. 2000. An empirical examination of self-reported work stress among U.S. managers. *J Appl Psychol* 85(1):65–74.

Chen, W. Q., O. L. Siu, J. F. Lu, C. L. Cooper, and D. R. Phillips. 2009. Work stress and depression: The direct and moderating effects of informal social support and coping. *Stress Health* 25(5):431–443.

Clays, E., D. De Bacquer, F. Leynen, M. Kornitzer, F. Kittel, and G. De Backer. 2007. Job stress and depression symptoms in middle-aged workers: Prospective results from the Belstress study. *Scand J Work Environ Health* 33(4):4252–4259.

Consedine, N. S. 2008. Health-promoting and health-damaging effects of emotions: The view from developmental functionalism. In *Handbook of emotions*, 3 ed., eds. M. Lewis, J. M. Haviland-Jones, and L. F. Barrett, 676–690. New York: Guilford Press.

de Beer, L. T., J. Pienaar, and S. Rothmann. 2016. Work overload, burnout, and psychological ill-health symptoms: A three-wave mediation model of the employee health impairment process. *Anxiety Stress Coping* 29(4):387–399.

Demerouti, E., A. B. Bakker, F. Nachreiner, and W. B. Schaufeli. 2001. The job demands-resources model of burnout. *J Appl Psychol* 86(3):499–512.

Ekman, P. 1973. *Darwin and facial expression: A century of research in review*. New York: Academic Press.

Ekstedt, M., M. Söderström, T. Åkerstedt, J. Nilsson, H. P. Søndergaard, and P. Alexander. 2006. Disturbed sleep and fatigue in occupational burnout. *Scand J Work Environ Health* 32(2):121–131.

Ferrari, A. J., F. J. Charlson, R. E. Norman, and S. B. Patten. 2013. Burden of depressive disorders by country, sex, age, and year: Findings from the global burden of disease study 2010. *PLoS Med* 10:1–12.

Gross, J. J. 1989. Emotion expression in cancer onset and progression. *Soc Sci Med* 28(12):1239–1248.

Hakanen, J., A. B. Bakker, and W. B. Schaufeli. 2006. Burnout and work engagement among teachers. *J School Psychol* 43(6):495–513.

Hakanen, J. J., W. B. Schaufeli, and K. Ahola. 2008. The job demands-resources model: A three-year cross-lagged study of burnout, depression, commitment and work engagement. *Work Stress* 22(3):224–241.

Hasenfeld, Y. 1974. *Human service organisations: A book of readings*. Ann Arbor: University of Michigan Press.

Heuven, E., A. B. Bakker, W. B. Schaufeli, and N. Huisman. 2006. The role of self-efficacy in performing emotion work. *J Vocat Behav* 69(2):222–235.

Hobfoll, S. E. 1989. Conservation of resources: A new attempt at conceptualizing stress. *Am Psychol* 44(3):513–524.

Hochschild, A. 1983. *The managed heart: Commercialization of human feeling*. Berkeley: University of California Press.

Hockey, G. J. 1997. Compensatory control in the regulation of human performance under stress and high workload: A cognitive – energetical framework. *Biol Psychol* 45(1–3):73–93.

Hu, Q., W. B. Schaufeli, and T. W. Taris. 2011. The job demands-resources model: An analysis of additive and joint effects of demands and resources. *J Vocat Behav* 79(1):181–190.

Idris, M. A., M. F. Dollard, and Yulita. 2014. Psychosocial safety climate, emotional demands, burnout, and depression: A longitudinal multilevel study in the Malaysian private sector. *J Occup Health Psychol* 19(3):291–302.

Jex, S. M., and P. D. Bliese. 1999. Efficacy beliefs as a moderator of the impact of work-related stressors: A multilevel study. *J Appl Psychol* 84(3):349–361.

Karasek, R. A. 1979. Job demands, job decision latitude and mental strain: Implications for job redesign. *Adm Sci Q* 24(2):285–308.

Karasek, R. A., and T. Theorell. 1990. *Healthy work: Stress, productivity and the reconstruction of working life.* New York: Basic Books.

Kemeny, M. E., and A. Shestyuk. 2008 Emotions, the neuroendocrine and immune systems, and health. In *Handbook of emotions*, 3 ed., eds. M. Lewis, J. M. Haviland-Jones, and L. F. Barrett, 661–675. New York: Guilford Press.

Kim, I. H., S. Noh, and C. Muntaner. 2013. Emotional demands and the risks of depression among homecare workers in the USA. *Int Arch Occup Environ Health* 86(6): 635–644.

Kline, R. B. 2011. *Principles and practices of structural equation modelling.* New York: Guilford Press.

Lee, R. T., and B. E. Ashforth. 1996. A meta-analytic examination of the correlates of the three dimensions of job burnout. *J Appl Psychol* 81(2):123–133.

Lewig, K. A., D. Xanthopoulou, A. B. Bakker, M. F. Dollard, and J. C. Metzer. 2007. Burnout and connectedness among Australian volunteers: A test of the job demands–resources model. *J Vocat Behav* 71(3):429–445.

Lorente Prieto, L., M. Salanova, M. I. M. Martínez, and W. B. Schaufeli. 2008. Extension of the job demands-resources model in the prediction of burnout and engagement among teachers over time. *Psicothema* 20(3):354–360.

Madsen, I. E. H., F. Diderichsen, H. Burr, and R. Rugulies. 2010. Person-related work and incident use of antidepressants: Relations and mediating factors from the Danish work environment cohort study. *Scand J Work Environ Health* 36(6):435–444.

Madsen, I. E. H., S. T. Nyberg, L. L. Magnusson Hanson et al. 2017. Job strain as a risk factor for clinical depression: Systematic review and meta-analysis with additional individual participant data. *Psychol Med* 47(8):1342–1356.

Magnusson Hanson, L. L., I. E. Madsen, H. Westerlund, T. Theorell, H. Burr, and R. Rugulies. 2013. Antidepressant use and associations with psychosocial work characteristics: A comparative study of Swedish and Danish gainfully employed. *J Affect Disord* 149(1–3):38–45.

Mäkikangas, A., and U. Kinnunen. 2003. Psychosocial work Stressors and well-being: Self-esteem and optimism as moderators in a one-year longitudinal sample. *Pers Individ Dif* 35(3):537–557.

Maxwell, S. E., D. A. Cole, and M. A. Mitchell. 2011. Bias in cross-sectional analyses of longitudinal mediation: Partial and complete mediation under an autoregressive model. *Multivariate Behav Res* 46(5):816–841.

Mayne, T. 2001. Emotions and health. In *Emotions: Currrent issues and future directions*, eds. T. J. Mayne, and G. A. Bonanno, 361–397. New York: Guilford Press.

Melamed, S., A. Shirom, S. Toker, and I. Shapira. 2006. Burnout and risk of type 2 diabetes: A prospective study of apparently healthy employed persons. *Psychosom Med* 68(6):863–869.

Melamed, S., U. Ugarten, A. Shirom, L. Kahana, Y. Lerman, and P. Froom. 1999. Chronic burnout, somatic arousal and elevated salivary cortisol levels. *J Psychosom Res* 46:591–598.

Moffitt, T. E., A. Caspi, and A. Taylor. 2010. How common are common mental disorders? Evidence that lifetime prevalence rates are doubled by prospective versus retrospective ascertainment. *Psychol Med* 40(6):899–909.

Moskowitz, J. T. 2001. Emotion and coping. In *Emotions: Currrent issues and future directions*, eds. T. J. Mayne, and G. A. Bonanno, 311–336. New York: Guilford Press.

Muntaner, C., Y. Li, X. Xue, T. Thompson, H. Chung, and P. O'Campo. 2006. County and organizational predictors of depression symptoms among low-income nursing assistants in the USA. *Soc Sci Med* 63(6):1454–1465.

Netterstrøm, B., N. Conrad, P. Bech et al. 2008. The relation between work-related psychosocial factors and the development of depression. *Epidemiol Rev* 30:118–132.

Niedhammer, I., L. Malard, and J. F. Chastang. 2015. Occupational factors and subsequent major depressive and generalized anxiety disorders in the prospective French national SIP study. *BMC Public Health* 15:200.

Nieuwenhuijsen, K., D. Bruinvels, and M. Frings-Dresen. 2010. Psychosocial work environment and stress-related disorders: A systematic review. *Occup Med* 60:277–286.

Pejtersen, J. H., T. S. Kristensen, and V. Borg. 2010. The second version of the Copenhagen Psychosocial Questionnaire. *Scand J Public Health* 38(Suppl. 3):8–24.

Plaisier, I., J. G. de Bruijn, R. de Graaf, M. ten Have, A. T. Beekman, and B. W. Penninx. 2007. The contribution of working conditions and social support to the onset of depressive and anxiety disorders among male and female employees. *Soc Sci Med* 64(2):401–410.

Radloff, L. S. 1977. The CES-D Scale: A self-report depression scale for research in the general population. *Appl Psychol Meas* 1(3):385–401.

Rothmann, S., and N. Essenko. 2007. Job characteristics, optimism, burnout, and ill health of support staff in a higher education institution in South Africa. *S Afr J Psychol* 37(1):135–152.

Rucker, D. D., K. J. Preacher, Z. L. Tormala, and R. E. Petty. 2011. Mediation analysis in social psychology: Current practices and new recommendations. *Soc Personal Psychol Compass* 5–6:359–371.

Rugulies, R. A. B., and I. E. H. Madsen. 2017. Effort–reward imbalance at work and risk of depressive disorders. A systematic review and meta-analysis of prospective cohort studies. *Scand J Work Environ Health* 43(4):294–306.

Schaufeli, W. B., and A. B. Bakker. 2004. Job demands, job resources and their relationship with burnout and engagement: A multi-sample study. *J Organ Behav* 25:293–315.

Sharma, S. 1996. *Applied multivariate techniques*. New York: John Willey & Sons.

Shields, M. 2006. Stress and depression in the employed population. *Health Rep* 17(4):11–29.

Siegrist, J. 2008. Chronic psychosocial stress at work and risk of depression: Evidence from prospective studies. *Eur Arch Psychiatry Clin Neurosci* 258(Suppl. 5):115–119.

Sobel, M. E. 1982. Asymptotic intervals for indirect effects in structural equations models. In *Sociological methodology*, ed. S. Leinhart, 290–312. San Francisco, CA: Jossey-Bass.

Soderfeldt, B., M. Soderfeldt, C. Muntaner, P. O'Campo, L. E. Warg, and C. G. Ohlson. 1996. Psychosocial work environment in human service organizations: A conceptual analysis and development of the demand-control model. *Soc Sci Med* 42(9):1217.

Steadman, K., and T. Taskila. 2015. *Symptoms of depression and their effects on employment*. The Work Foundation. http://www.theworkfoundation.com/wp-content/uploads/2016/11/382_Symptoms-of-Depression_FINAL.pdf (accessed November 3, 2019).

Sundin, L., J. Hochwalder, C. Bildt, and J. Lisspers. 2007. The relationship between different work-related sources of social support and burnout among registered and assistant nurses in Sweden: A questionnaire survey. *Int J Nurse Stud* 44(5):758–769.

Szczygieł, D., and Ł. Baka. 2016. The role of personal resources in the relationship between job stressors and job burnout. *Polish J Appl Psychol* 14(2):133–152.

Theorell, T., A. Hammarström, G. Aronsson et al. 2015. A systematic review including meta-analysis of work environment and depressive symptoms. *BMC Public Health* 15:738.

Tremblay, M. A., and D. Messervey. 2011. The job demands-resources model: Further evidence for the buffering effect of personal resources. *J Ind Psychol* 37(2):10–19.

van den Heuvel, M., E. Demerouti, and W. B. Schaufeli. 2010. Personal resources and work engagement in the face of change. In *Contemporary occupational health psychology: Global perspectives on research and practice*, eds. J. I. Houdmont, and S. Leka, 124–150. Chichester: John Wiley & Sons Ltd.

Van Maanen, J., and G. Kunda. 1989. Real feelings: Emotional expression and organizational culture. *Res Organ Behav* 11:43–103.

van Vegchel, N., J. de Jonge, M. Söderfeldt, C. Dormann, and W. Schaufeli. 2004. Quantitative versus emotional demands among Swedish human service employees: Moderating effects of job control and social support. *Int J Stress Manag* 11(1):21–40.

Van Yperen, N. W., and T. A. Snijders. 2000. A multilevel analysis of the demands-control model. Is stress at work determined by factors at the group level or individual level? *J Occup Health Psychol* 5(1):182–190.

Whiteford, H. A., L. Degenhardt, J. Rehm et al. 2013. Global burden of disease attributable to mental and substance use disorders: Findings from the global burden of disease study 2010. *Lancet* 382(9904):1575–1586.

Wieclaw, J., E. Agerbo, P. Bo Mortensen, H. Burr, F. Tuchsen, and J. Bonde. 2008. Psychosocial working conditions and the risk of depression and anxiety disorders in the Danish workforce. *BMC Public Health* 8(1):280–290.

Williams, J., and D. P. MacKinnon. 2008. Resampling and distribution of the product methods for testing indirect effects in complex models. *Struct Equ Modeling* 15(1):23–51.

Wittchen, H. U., F. Jacobi, J. Rehm et al. 2010. The size and burden of mental disorders and other disorders of the brain in Europe 2010. *Eur Neuropsychopharmacol* 21(9):655–679.

Xanthopolou, D., A. B. Bakker, and W. B. Schaufeli. 2007. The role of personal resources in the job-resources model. *Int J Stress Manag* 14(2):121–141.

Zapf, D. 2002. Emotion work and psychological well-being: A review of the literature and some conceptual considerations. *Hum Res Manag Rev* 12(2):237–268.

Żołnierczyk-Zreda, D., and P. Holas. 2018. Psychosocial working conditions and major depression or depressive disorders: Review of studies. *Med Pr* 69(5):573–581.

5 Determinants and Consequences of Work-Related Stress in Personnel of Residential Care Establishments

Andrzej Najmiec

CONTENTS

5.1   INTRODUCTION

The aim of this chapter is to examine the basic sources of stress and its health consequences among personnel of residential care establishments, caring for residents with various chronic mental illnesses and for intellectually disabled children, adolescents, or adults in Poland. The practical outcome of the study is to propose a variety of stress-coping support programs, effectively helping to cope with work-related stress experienced by this occupational group.

The paper has been prepared at the Central Institute of Labour Protection – National Research Institute in Warsaw, Poland, on the basis of a research project, entitled *Stress management support programs for persons performing selected special character jobs*, and its results. The special character jobs are defined as occupations requiring particular responsibilities and psychophysical fitness, the ability of which to be properly performed without endangering public safety, including the health or life of others, is reduced before reaching the retirement age as a result of deteriorating psychophysical fitness associated with the aging process [Dz.U 2008].

The project covered a total of 601 persons of three special character professional groups, including 200 employees of residential care establishments, and was conducted in the period from May to July 2017 in residential care homes located in all 16 voivodships of Poland.

The physical and mental health status, lifestyle and psychosocial working conditions of residential care workers have been described in terms of both stress-inducing and health improving factors. The research results have shown that the main cause of stress at work for the residential care employee group is high job demands related to emotional stress and low skill development opportunities. Health problems revealed in this occupational group, including mainly back pain, may be a consequence of physical strain at work (lifting patients), stress, as well as a lack of physical exercise during leisure time. The physical inactivity factor may result from occupational stress and physical strain and contribute to a reduced ability to cope with stress at work.

The proposed stress management support programs are built on the residential care employee group research results and the identified occupational stressors. Personal and organizational measures have been considered in the development of the support schemes. The study authors hope that these programs and other research findings presented in this chapter will help managers and OSH specialists in shaping psychosocial working conditions, through supporting residential care workers in performing their difficult and responsible work with greater satisfaction, while maintaining a healthy work–life balance.

5.2   THE WORK OF RESIDENTIAL CARE ESTABLISHMENT PERSONNEL

Residential care homes are one of the most important and numerous social support institutions in Poland. The assistance involves 24-hour or day care provided to persons who are unable to live independently or whose permanent residences cannot be adapted to their needs to enable independent living; these limitations result from the age, disease, living conditions, family situation, housing, or material conditions of the patient, despite all the available forms of assistance used [Lalak and Pilch 1996]. Diverse organizational settings of residential care homes correspond to the public, non-governmental and private care establishments. The mission of residential care homes is to provide living, caring, supporting, and educational services according to set standards and individual needs of the residents.

Housing needs include, first and foremost: 1) ensuring an adequate place of residence without architectural barriers hindering transport, 2) food and meal preparation, and 3) maintaining clean spaces. The provision of care is based on assistance in dealing with personal matters, basic life activities, personal hygiene, and supply of personal hygiene products. Residential care homes are also charged with organizing the work of therapeutic and social care teams, as well as providing various social support services such as:

- community work opportunities
- services addressed to residents:
    - occupational therapy,
    - access to library and daily press,
    - arts and culture events,
    - regular contact with the general manager,
    - efficient handling of complaints and requests,
    - ensuring conditions for the development of self-governance among home residents,
    - access to psychological consultations/therapy,
    - assisting in religious practices,
    - ensuring safe storage of money and valuables,
    - funeral services according to the deceased resident's practiced faith.

Residential care homes for children and young people with intellectual disabilities also provide educational services, enabling the younger residents to participate in education, social rehabilitation workshops, and learning through life experiences.

Residential care homes, depending on the resident group, are divided into the following categories of residents:

- elderly,
- chronically somatically ill persons,
- chronically mentally ill persons,
- adults with intellectual disabilities,
- persons with physical disabilities,
- alcohol addicts.

Currently employed at residential care homes are social workers, educators, psychologists, occupational therapists, care workers, nurses, and physiotherapists. An effective implementation of care and support services is subject to the full-time employment of social workers and their access to psychologist consultations.

5.3 WORK-RELATED STRESS AMONG WORKERS CARING FOR PATIENTS OF RESIDENTIAL CARE HOMES

The specific nature of the work performed by the occupational groups working with specific categories of clients/patients in residential care homes (*staff caring for residents of residential care homes for chronically mentally ill and mentally disabled persons*) exposes them to a number of stressors, including difficult and hazardous situations. Stress sources in this occupational group may result from their relationship with residents, psychosocial working conditions, the physical working environment, and physical strain.

Direct reports by personnel of residential care homes describing the risks, such as "I was exposed to physical attacks from the residents during my employment [...] I was beaten once by a mentally ill person", as well as media reports, show that aggression, violence, and other confrontational behaviors are not uncommon in residential care homes, and that they can take many different forms, from verbal aggression to active violence. It is unlikely to find a residential care establishment where at least a few residents would not be inclined, or would not tend, to be periodically aggressive. Violent behavior may be caused not only by age-specific factors and diseases, but also by factors related to the functioning of the residential care home. Patients may notice that they gradually have less control over their own lives and that other persons, including the staff, decide for them the course of their day and the activities they perform. Aggression in this case is mostly a form of reaction aimed at strengthening one's own position. Violent behavior can be manifested by new residents who find themselves in the care facility against their will. In such situations, aggression can be a result of disappointment and a sense of rejection by loved ones. In turn, assisting these often so-called difficult residents, as well as the accompanying stress and overwork, poor job satisfaction, low social and professional status, high job demands, and low remuneration, exacerbate the risk of emotional exhaustion among personnel of residential care homes.

A study aimed at investigating the well-being of residential care workers and their attitude toward work was conducted among residential care staff employed in hostels, night shelters, community care centers, social integration centers, and specialist establishments. [Rymsza 2012]. All respondent groups indicated the low social status of their profession, however, the prevailing group in this respect were social care workers. Those respondents were the least satisfied with the remuneration for the work. The specialist establishment social workers declared the lowest salaries, but were also more satisfied with the remuneration they received than other surveyed groups. They also reported the lowest stress levels, the highest being noted among residential care workers. Similarly, the latter group experienced job burnout syndrome more frequently than all other respondents.

Another research study conducted among residential care workers [Szmagalski 2009] examined the extent to which employees were exposed to job burnout and the correlating factors. Among the problems most frequently raised by the surveyed workers were the low social status of the profession, the constant and routine contact with residents, being overqualified, performing unskilled work, the low wages, and the stressful working environment. The following were also mentioned:

poor job satisfaction (low work outcomes), unsatisfied residents, and lack of career development opportunities. The main factors accompanying job burnout were poor emotion coping skills and low individual predispositions for social work or caring roles. Such conditions led to depersonalization, disengagement from work, and disconnection from the residents manifested in an indifferent attitude and labeling of residents.

Moreover, an analysis of studies carried out among various groups of social workers [Fengler 2001] revealed other characteristics of the working conditions that also correlated with job burnout. These were:

- excessive responsibility, no recognition of effort, ineffective communication, poor satisfaction with management,
- job demands, lack of social support,
- frequent changes in resident care instructions, no influence on the allocation of residents, previous alcohol addiction,
- poor job satisfaction, increased alcohol and drug consumption, constant search for another job, number of sick leaves, poor due diligence,
- unresolved interpersonal conflicts, unrealistic earnings expectations, conflicts between personal and institutional goals, and structural difficulties at the institution.

Recent studies in groups of social workers show different relationships between working conditions and mental health. In a study conducted in the United States in a group of over 100 nurses working in residential care homes at different job seniority levels [Zhang et al. 2016], mental health was associated with different working conditions in different nurse groups: physical safety and work–home conflict among the nursing assistants, work–home conflict among the licensed practical nurses, and physical job demands among the registered nurses.

Relationships between occupational stress, social support, and burnout were studied in a group of long-term care nursing staff [Woodhead, Northrop, and Edelstein 2014]. The results revealed that job demands (greater occupational stress) were associated with greater emotional exhaustion depersonalization, and a lesser personal accomplishment. Social support at work as well as family support were associated with reduced emotional exhaustion and higher levels of personal accomplishment.

In addition to work-related variables (workload and burnout), studies among nursing home professionals have revealed that the level of anxiety of workers is associated with patients' family members and their feelings of guilt arising from limited care possibilities [Gallego-Alberto et al. 2018].

Studies conducted in a Polish group of palliative care nurses [Ogińska-Bulik 2018] have shown that nurses working in palliative care experience the negative consequences of stress at work, i.e. burnout and secondary traumatic stress, which are interrelated. Disengagement from work has been found to increase the risk of secondary traumatic stress. The practical conclusion of the research has been that measures supporting work-related stress – coping skills and developing personal and social resources – are vital.

5.4 STUDY GROUP

The project study sample included three distinct, special character job groups:

- G1 – teachers, educators and other teaching staff employed in youth education centers, youth rehabilitation centers, education centers, youth hostels, and youth correctional facilities ($n = 200$),
- G2 – personnel caring for patients of residential care homes for chronically mentally ill or mentally disabled children and adolescents or adults ($n = 200$),
- G3 – medical staff of psychiatric wards and addiction treatment in direct contact with the patient ($n = 201$).

In the G2 group, women prevailed, with $n = 179$ (89.5%), while for men $n = 21$ persons (10.5%). The age of the respondents was between 20 and 63 years, and the mean age was $M = 42.2$ ($SD = 9.71$). The largest number of respondents had completed higher education (53.8%) and secondary education (24.6%). The mean career length in the occupation was $M = 13.2$ years ($SD = 8.99$). The G2 group respondents were employed in the following types of institutions:

- residential care homes (126 persons),
- social care centers (17 persons),
- community care centers (14 persons),
- social care centers for the mentally ill (12 persons),
- veteran residential care homes (9 persons),
- social care foundations (6 persons),
- residential care homes for the chronically mentally ill (6 persons),
- residential care homes for adults with intellectual disabilities (4 persons),
- residential care homes for the mentally ill (3 persons),
- residential care homes for children and youth with intellectual disabilities (3 persons).

The majority of the G2 group were employed as occupational therapists (18%), social workers (10.5%), nurses (10%), and ward nurses (7.0%). The remaining respondents were psychologists (ten persons), educators (five persons), paramedics (four persons), a teacher, and an addiction therapist. In the G2 group, 90% were state-employed persons. The percentage share of manual and white-collar workers in the G2 group was nearly equal (39% and 40.5% respectively). A mix of manual and intellectual work was declared by 18% of the G2 group respondents.

The special character of residential care work is the intense and direct contact with patients, coupled with provision of assistance in various forms, from saving lives and health care duties, to constant care for the sick and elderly.

The sample selection was carried out using the quota sampling method, taking into account the age and gender structure of each institution where the research was conducted.

5.5 METHOD

The Copenhagen Psychosocial Questionnaire II (COPSOQ) long version was used to assess the psychosocial working conditions and quality of life of the respondents [COPSOQ II 2007]. The COPSOQ II questionnaire has been increasingly used to study psychosocial working conditions and has therefore been translated into many languages, including English, Chinese, Japanese, Flemish, Spanish, Portuguese, German, and Polish. The questionnaire consists of 41 scales with 127 items and includes the following work-related aspects:

- job demands (18 items): quality demands, cognitive demands, emotional demands, work pace, hiding emotions demands,
- work organization and content (17 items): job control, skill development opportunities, task diversification, importance of work, work engagement,
- social relations and leadership (22 items): recognition at work, predictability of work, role clarity, role conflict, co-worker social support, management social support, leadership quality, social relations,
- work-to-home relationship (17 items): work-to-home conflict, home-to-work conflict, job security, job satisfaction,
- values at work (15 items): trust between co-workers, management trust in employees, fairness, social inclusion,
- health and well-being in the last 4 weeks (31 items): general health, sleep problems, burnout, stress, depression symptoms, somatic stress, physical and mental stress symptoms, coping problems,
- exposure to unwanted conduct in the last 12 months (7 items): sexual harassment, threat of violence, physical violence, harassment, workplace bullying, conflicts and quarrels, gossip and false accusations.

The psychometric properties of the questionnaire are satisfactory. The internal consistency calculated for eight selected scales has been satisfactory (Cronbach's $\alpha = 0.75$-0.85) for seven scales. In turn, research on the reliability of COPSOQ II medium version, extended by an additional 25 items (112 items in total), conducted in a group of 349 Danish workers using the intra-group correlation (interclass correlation – ICC) method, has shown a satisfactory reliability (0.70–0.89), except for the *trust between co-workers* items.

The study was conducted in the period from May to July 2017. The study covered 35 establishments located in all 16 voivodships of Poland.

5.6 STUDY RESULTS

5.6.1 Health Status

The residential care home employee group has been subjectively characterized by a good health condition. The vast majority of respondents (85.8%) assessed their health as *good*, *very good* and *excellent*. The self-assessment of health status is shown in Figure 5.1.

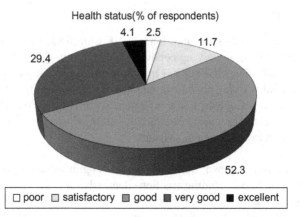

FIGURE 5.1   Self-assessment of health status in the residential care home employee group.

Taking into account 14 types of diseases analyzed, the vast majority of employees had never suffered from them and almost half of respondents (45.6%) had not taken sick leave during the 12 months preceding the survey. However, the ailment most frequently mentioned by the surveyed residential care workers was back pain (24.2%), followed by hypertension (14.5%) and allergies (9.8%). The majority of respondents *rarely* or *never* took sedatives or sleeping pills, but much more often used analgesics (49.2% of respondents). Figure 5.2 shows the prevalence of individual disease among the surveyed residential care workers.

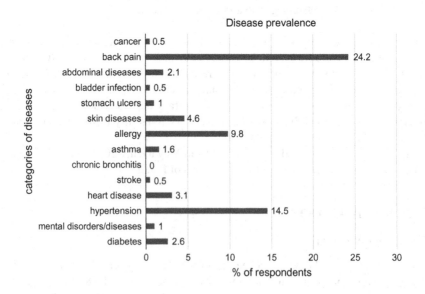

FIGURE 5.2   Frequency of disease incidence among the residential care home staff.

5.6.2 Lifestyle

The residential care home staff practiced a rather healthy lifestyle: the vast majority did not smoke cigarettes (75.1%), but more than 15% of respondents smoked 10 or more cigarettes a day. The majority of respondents declared abstinence from alcohol.

In terms of physical activity, the largest group of workers (42.5%) undertook light activity for 2–4 hours a week (e.g. walking, light gardening work, light exercising, etc.), and around 30% declared an intensive activity (e.g. fast walking, cycling at high speed or other high-sweat cardio exercises) for 2–4 hours a week. The least numerous group (4.5%) opted for an intense physical activity for more than 4 hours a week or regular, heavy exercises/training sessions. However, a worrying phenomenon was the fact that 23.5% of respondents were physically inactive after work, spending leisure time on reading newspapers or books, or watching television. This could have been caused by a significant physical strain at work and musculoskeletal ailments (mainly back pain). Musculoskeletal disorders and the lack of physical activity after work could have significantly reduced these workers' ability to cope with stress.

5.6.3 Mental Health Status

The vast majority of respondents in the four weeks preceding the survey had not had any sleeping problems (they had fallen asleep easily and had not woken up during the night).

Frequent incidence of depression symptoms (classed as *most of the time* or *always*) was found in a small percentage of the study group: feeling sad (7.5%), lacking self-confidence (7.5%), remorse or guilt (5%), and lack of interest in everyday matters (3.5%).

Respondents usually did not feel symptoms of cognitive stress – there was observed a rare incidence of concentration and memory problems, or difficulties with clear thinking, and decision making. The symptoms of somatic stress, such as headaches, stomach problems, heart palpitations, and persisting muscle tension were also low.

More than half of respondents felt symptoms of psychological stress such as resting problems and tension *rarely* or *not at all*, but almost 15% of respondents admitted that they felt stressed *often* or *all the time*.

It is worth noting the problem of professional burnout. Although around 45% of respondents felt symptoms of this phenomenon *rarely* or *not at all*, a significant percentage complained about *frequent* or *persistent* feelings of lack of strength (13.6%), physical exhaustion (16.7%), emotional exhaustion (10.5%), and general fatigue (18.0%).

Figures 5.3 and 5.4 show the severity of depression and burnout symptoms in the surveyed group of residential care home staff.

5.6.4 Psychosocial Working Conditions

In terms of psychosocial working conditions, the residential care workers rated *emotional demands* highly: more than 72% of respondents believed that professional

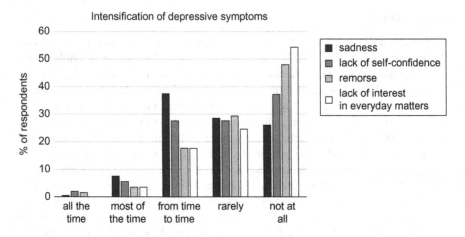

FIGURE 5.3 Intensification of depressive symptoms among the residential care home employee group.

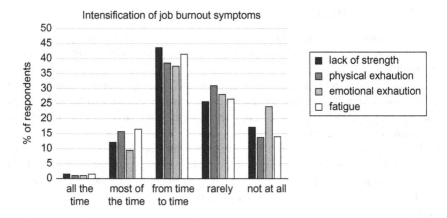

FIGURE 5.4 Intensification of job burnout symptoms among the residential care home employee group.

duties *always* or *often* required addressing other people's problems, and more than 73% of respondents believed that work was emotionally demanding. Nearly half of respondents in this occupational group were of an opinion that their work *always* or *often* put them in emotionally difficult situations. This aspect of work could be a significant burden for workers and therefore necessitates action to improve workers' ability to cope with emotional strain. Figure 5.5 illustrates the level of different aspects of emotional demands among the residential care home employee group.

An adverse aspect of the psychosocial working conditions experienced by residential care home workers has been the low personal development prospects. Nearly 30% of the surveyed workers in this professional group claimed that they did not have an opportunity to develop their skills at work and about 20% of respondents believed that they did not have a chance to learn new competences.

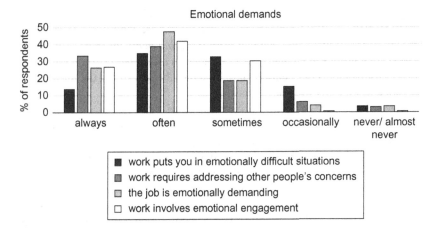

FIGURE 5.5   Emotional demands in the residential care home employee group.

Another important negative aspect has been the exposure to unwanted conduct. Figure 5.6 illustrates the scale of this phenomenon. Although the majority of respondents had not experienced unwanted conduct (from 54.5% who had not experienced *gossip or false accusations* to 94.5% who had not experienced *unwanted sexual interest*) in the 12 months preceding the survey, all these behaviors had occurred at least several times during that time.

The most common form of unwanted conduct among the residential care home employee group was *gossip and false accusations*, which affected 45.5%

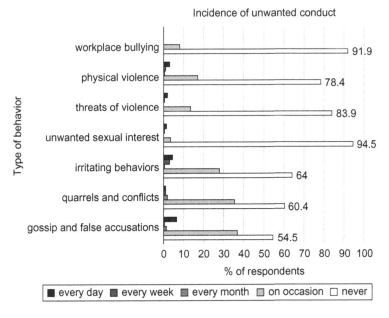

FIGURE 5.6   Frequency of exposure to unwanted conduct among the residential care home employee group.

of respondents, as well as *quarrels and conflicts* which was experienced by about 40% of employees. The source of these behaviors were mainly co-workers. Other dominant forms of unwanted conduct were *irritating behavior* (36%), *physical violence* (21.6%), *threats of violence* (16.1%), and even *unwanted sexual interest* (5.5%), received from patients or clients Figure 5.7 shows the severity of the unwanted conduct incidence, highlighting its sources.

The residential care home workers are characterized by the meaning they ascribe to their work. About 83% of the surveyed workers were convinced that their work was *important* and 53% of respondents were *highly* or *very* motivated and engaged at work. The vast majority of respondents believed that they were aware of the purpose of their work (70.7%) and the responsibility entrusted to them (77.5%).

Despite the aforementioned strenuous interpersonal relations at work, nearly 80% of respondents believed that the social climate was *always* good (24.6%) or *often* good (54.9%) and over 70% felt part of the community in the workplace (Figure 5.8). The vast majority of the surveyed employees felt satisfied with their work: 70% of employees were *satisfied* or *very satisfied* with their job prospects, and over 74% were satisfied with their physical working conditions. The respondents were unlikely to be afraid of losing their jobs: 72% of respondents were not worried about being dismissed and 65.5% did not fear being transferred to another position against their will.

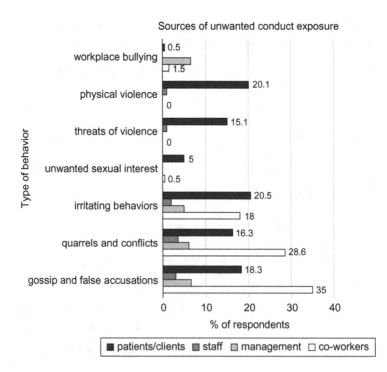

FIGURE 5.7 Sources of exposure to unwanted conduct among the residential care home employee group.

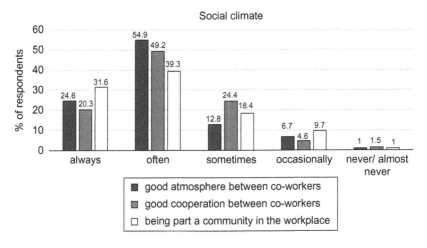

FIGURE 5.8 Social climate among the residential care home employees.

Around 97% of respondents believed that time spent on family life had *little* or *no* negative impact on their professional career, but much less (around 81%) believed that time spent on work did not affect family life. A similar assessment concerned the negative impact of effort invested at work and in private life.

5.7 SUMMARY OF THE RESIDENTIAL CARE HOME EMPLOYEE GROUP SURVEY RESULTS

5.7.1 Job Demands

The residential care home workers, similar to the previously discussed occupational group, are characterized by a slow work pace and high emotional demands. The slow work pace is certainly a significant psychosocial working conditions asset, as it means that there is no need to carry out professional tasks under strong time pressure and in a constant hurry during the working shift. However, high emotional demands, coupled with the need to act and function professionally in emotionally difficult situations, which require attention and emotional engagement in the personal problems of patients, should be considered as a vulnerability.

5.7.2 Work Organization and Content

The residential care home employees rate personal development opportunities as low. It thus seems that there are significantly fewer opportunities for this occupational group to act on their own initiative, use their skills and expertise at work, learn new competences, and develop human capital compared to the other two groups surveyed. This result should be counted among the poor psychosocial working conditions of residential care home workers and as a potential source of stress.

5.7.3   HEALTH AND WELL-BEING

Among the residential care home employees, there was a significantly higher percentage of employees complaining of musculoskeletal disorders (back pain) compared to the other two occupational groups (medical personnel of psychiatric wards and youth rehabilitation professionals). Moreover, the highest percentage in the residential care home employee group, out of all the three occupational groups surveyed, admitted to physical inactivity during leisure time. Musculoskeletal disorders and reduced physical activity after work can significantly reduce the ability of the residential care home employees to cope with occupational stress.

In comparison to the Danish studies, the following factors can be considered negative working conditions of residential care home employees:

- high emotional demands,
- lower personal development opportunities,
- higher percentage of persons complaining of musculoskeletal disorders (back pain),
- higher percentage of persons physically inactive.

5.8   WORK-RELATED STRESS MANAGEMENT SUPPORT PROGRAM FOR THE PERSONNEL OF RESIDENTIAL CARE ESTABLISHMENTS

Workplace-based research has shown that excessive job demands, poor job control, low social support, and other psychosocial factors create a risk of stress reactions which, if frequent or prolonged, lead to a deterioration in the physical and mental well-being of the worker, alongside many other health conditions [Łuczak and Żołnierczyk-Zreda 2002]. In turn, the ability to cope with stress prevents or minimizes these negative impacts at the individual level.

A study carried out by Cameron and Brownie [2010] has attempted to identify the factors that affect mental resilience in nurses caring for the elderly, namely their adaptive, physical, mental, and emotional abilities, which are required for this type of work. Nine nurses working in retirement homes on the Sunshine Coast in Queensland were examined. They were asked to reflect on the phenomenon of resilience in the workplace. The study showed that clinical experience, a sense of purpose in a comprehensive (holistic) care environment, positive attitudes, and a work–life balance were important determinants of resilience observed in nurses caring for the elderly. Maintaining long-lasting, meaningful relationships with patients, receiving co-worker support, and adopting a humorous approach to stress relief were conducive to well-being and mental resilience in the workplace.

A qualitative study by Ablett and Jones [2007] examined the factors that supported mental resilience and well-being among palliative care workers. To describe the experiences of hospice nurses, interpretative phenomenological analysis (IPA) was used. It included motives concerning interpersonal factors that influenced nurses' decisions to start and continue working in palliative care, and their attitude toward life and work. The emerging motives were compared with theoretical constructs of personalities and a sense of coherence. The comparison revealed many similarities. The nurses manifested a high level of engagement and attributed a sense of purpose to their work. The study group differed in terms of their reaction to change, and this was discussed in relation to stress resilience and a sense of coherence. Implications for the well-being of palliative care workers, and training and support programs that could have an impact on the quality of patient care, were also discussed.

Furthermore, stress can have a negative impact on the functioning of workers, including: work performance, sickness absence, job satisfaction, burnout, counterproductive work behavior, and employee turnover [e.g. Demerouti et al. 2001; Jensen, Patel, and Messersmith 2013; Baka 2017; Meisler, Vigoda-Gadot, and Drory 2017; Schonfeld, Bianchi, and Luehring-Jones 2017]. Hence, employers interested in improving worker health and minimizing health effects should take action to prevent stress at the workplace.

Workplace stress prevention should start with an assessment of the level and specificity of occupational stress, including a survey on the stress severity among workers and the identification of its sources. It is only after an initial assessment that changes should be introduced to the working environment to reduce stress levels and, where possible, eliminate stress sources and develop the employees' ability to cope with stress.

5.9   EMPLOYEE-ADDRESSED MEASURES

Stress prevention methods and efforts at limiting its consequences that are targeted at workers include, among others: participation in stress management programs, developing stress-coping skills, assertiveness, and promotion of a healthy lifestyle.

5.9.1   STRESS MANAGEMENT PROGRAMS

The current residential care home employee group study results have shown significant correlations ($p < 0.01$) between psychosocial working conditions and health and well-being indicators. The results have demonstrated that quantitative job demands significantly ($p < 0.01$) correlate with work–home conflict (Spearman's $\rho = 0.50$), depression (0.27), somatic (0.22) and cognitive stress (0.30). Therefore, workers should be given the opportunity to develop their psychological skills through participation in coping skills training sessions where they would learn how to cope with stress and practice relaxation techniques, as well as how to handle negative emotions and stress-inducing patient/client behavior. Equally vital are competence training sessions where skills such as time management, or how to cope with time pressure, are taught.

Participation in such stress management programs not only reduces perceived stress levels and depression symptoms while also improving one's ability to cope with difficult client/patient situations and with psychosocial stress, but it can also reduce blood pressure, boost positive attitude, and lead to a general improvement in mental health. Employee participation in this type of training may result in increased job satisfaction and improved performance [McCraty, Atkinson, and Tomasino 2003].

Among the many stress-coping techniques, it is worth mentioning:

- neuromuscular relaxation – consists in reducing mental tension through gradual, methodical muscle relaxation,
- breathing training – consists in learning deep diaphragm breathing and practicing focusing attention on the breathing process,
- MBSR (Mindfulness-Based Stress Reduction) – a stress reduction program based on focusing on current experience ("attention"). Scientific research has proven the effectiveness of MBSR in improving concentration skills, reducing stress, and increasing resilience to negative emotions [Grossman et al. 2004; Sharma and Rush 2014],
- cognitive-behavioral techniques – these are methods that combine the role of thought (attitude in developing motivation, and reactions) with behavioral change, e.g. cognitive assessment technique (teaches the individual to look at stressors from a different perspective) or cognitive tests technique (in simulated conditions, the individual learns about situations that usually cause anxiety in him/her, so that they are less stressful in real life).

5.9.2 Promoting Healthy Lifestyles

Physical activity not only improves physical health, but it also has a positive impact on mental well-being by developing self-confidence, optimism, and inner harmony, improving sleep quality, reducing anxiety and depression symptoms, and giving a sense of control over one's life [Mayo Clinic Staff 2018]. In the present study, a significant ($p < 0.01$) correlation between general health and sleeping problems has been identified in the group of residential care home workers (–0.34).

Healthy lifestyle factors that prevent the negative consequences of stress are:

- regular physical activity,
- proper nutrition,
- weight control,
- refraining from smoking and consuming alcohol,
- good quality sleep [Jones, Norman, and Wier 2010].

The current study results, in terms of healthy lifestyles among the residential care home employee group, have revealed the lowest consumption of beer and wine comparing to the other two occupational groups surveyed. Positive individual health habits are all the more important in the residential care home employee group as these workers have recorded the highest percentage of persons complaining of musculoskeletal disorders, especially back pain, and the highest percentage of persons remaining physically inactive during leisure time.

Healthy lifestyle programs, particularly physical activity, reduce sickness absenteeism, stress, and employee turnover, improve job satisfaction [Proper et al. 2002], and increase employee fitness, while also decreasing the occupational accident rate [Malińska, Namysł, and Hildt-Ciupińska 2012].

Employers can promote physical activity by creating exercise areas at the enterprise premises and providing short physical exercise breaks and bicycle parking spaces, or by supporting fitness or swimming club subscription plans, or organizing walking meetings, which is easier to implement in the case of residential care home premises with green areas surrounding the building or those located close to forest areas on city outskirts.

Other aspects of a healthy lifestyle can be addressed by providing regular preventive medical check-ups and allowing time for proper meal breaks, as well as promoting the integration and participation in activities of workers aged 50+.

In summary, the following support schemes can be introduced to reduce the risk of work-related stress among residential care home workers:

- introduction of a stress prevention program: monitoring, assessment and combating stress,
- ensuring employee participation in interpersonal training sessions covering communication skills and assertive behaviors,
- ensuring worker participation in stress management training – including stress induced by patient/client behavior,
- ensuring worker participation in management training sessions focused on anger- and stress-inducing patient/client behavior,
- enabling worker participation in time-management training sessions that enhance working under time pressure skills,
- promotion of a healthy lifestyle, including physical exercise, that helps in coping with emotions and stress,
- offering regular preventive medical check-ups,
- encouraging physical activity by facilitating access to different forms of activity, e.g. swimming pool tickets, gymnastics, excursions,
- provision of meal breaks and short physical exercise breaks during the working day,
- promoting the integration and undertaking of physical activities by employees aged 50+.

5.10 ORGANIZATION-ORIENTED ACTIVITIES

The launch of a stress prevention program should be preceded by a psychological diagnosis, including a periodic assessment of the psychosocial working conditions as well as an assessment of the mental and physical well-being of employees. To this end, various tools have been used to measure stressors at work and the consequences of stress, taking into account many comprehensive aspects of the working environment (e.g. the Copenhagen Questionnaire on Psychosocial Working Conditions – COPSOQ) or shorter questionnaires assessing the incidence of stress factors (e.g. the European Foundation for the Improvement of Working and Living Conditions – Eurofound questionnaire).

Previous research has proved that severe stress resulting from organizational factors is often experienced by persons working with patients or by those in an emotionally demanding social environment. This premise has been confirmed by the present study results, whereby organizational factors have been found to determine the level of job burnout: job burnout correlates significantly ($p < 0.01$) with the level of cognitive demands (Spearman's $\rho = 0.25$), emotional demands (0.20), work engagement (−0.20), leadership quality (−0.21) and the level of perceived organizational fairness and employee respect (−0.29). The high significance of leadership quality in the context of job burnout may indicate that preventive programs aimed at reducing the level of work-related stress should be supported by active participation of management in the implementation of such measures. Below are presented proposals for actions to reduce organizational limitations on activities related to work–home/home–work conflict that should reduce job burnout and have a positive impact on worker well-being, since job burnout ($p < 0.01$) correlates significantly with the assessment of work-to-home conflict (0.41). Each activity described below should be preceded by management training to raise awareness on the importance of these activities for the functioning of the organization, as well as to provide detailed procedures for their implementation.

5.10.1 Measures to Reduce Organizational Limitations at Work

The results of a survey conducted among various sectors' customer service employees [Mockałło and Najmiec 2017] present a number of possible actions aimed at reducing organizational limitations in working with patients. It is worth mentioning here, among others, the following projects, which relate to the residential care home occupational group:

- taking care of the workstation equipment (e.g. equipment reducing physical strain at work with patients) and providing staff with equipment-use training and ergonomic load lifting methods,
- reducing conflicting job demands (e.g. a demand to be empathic and not worry about patient complaints at the same time),
- limiting the "switching" from one activity to another, and avoiding a sudden allocation of random tasks, unless these activities are aimed at reducing the monotony of work,
- introducing procedures that promote job control and autonomy at work by increasing decision-making powers and introducing more flexible working hours where possible,
- ensuring fair treatment of all workers by enhancing the link between individual contributions at work and the rewards received, as well as a fair remuneration system and frequent (where possible) awarding of prizes, recognition, and distinctions,
- providing training to managers at all levels in order to familiarize the management with methods of reducing organizational limitations at work with a patient/client.

5.10.2 Measures to Reduce the Level of Job Demands

Based on research results obtained by Mockałło and Najmiec [2017], a number of actions can be identified that reduce the negative effect of excessive demands on employees when working with a patient/client, e.g.:

- reducing time pressure or the burden of new or urgent duties/tasks/responsibilities by: planning work in advance, scheduling activities with employees, informing employees in advance of planned shifts, reducing overtime and the need to work during leisure time,
- reducing the amount of work related to reporting and "bureaucracy", reducing the number of administrative duties, reducing the number of procedures as far as possible,
- adjusting the number of workers to the number of required personnel and undertaking actions aimed at preventing staff shortages,
- providing more flexible working time to reduce work–home conflict,
- adapting the amount of work to workers' capabilities (also in terms of age and experience) and enabling them to work at a pace adapted to their individual abilities and temperamental characteristics,
- increasing the participation of employees in the functioning of the organization by increasing worker participation in decision making and affording them more power and autonomy (e.g. at creating work schedules, allocating night shifts, selecting shift co-workers/partners),
- providing training to managers at all levels in order to familiarize management with methods of reducing quantitative demands and workload.

5.10.3 Actions to Prevent Stress-Inducing Patient/Client Behavior

In order to reduce stress-inducing patient/client behavior, procedures should be implemented to curb the negative consequences of such behaviors. This applies in particular to those occupational groups that work directly with patients/clients/customers. In an effort to contain this type of behavior, the organization should provide workers with periodic training on coping with hostile patient behavior, offering guidelines such as:

- allow the patient to vent her/his anger verbally without being interrupted,
- maintain visual contact,
- do not criticize the patient or this type of behavior at this point,
- do not embrace the patient's negative emotions,
- do not laugh at the patient,
- do not assume that the patient is motivated by hostile motives, but assume that he/she is explaining matters important to him/her,
- let it feel like you understand the patient's complaints,
- if possible, offer help.

When aggressive patient/client behavior is frequent, management should prepare, familiarize, and implement procedures to prevent it. These procedures should include, for example, rules for cooperation with security staff, covering staff procedures, security measures to increase the distance between staff and patients, etc.

5.10.4 Actions to Reduce Interpersonal Conflicts at Work

Interpersonal conflicts at work are an example of social demands relating to the quality of relations between workers. The essence of these is heavy interactions with managers and co-workers, at a varying degree of intensity – from minor quarrels to mental struggle [Spector and Jex 1998]. Interpersonal conflicts can take different forms – open (e.g. open criticism, depreciating comments) or hidden (e.g. spreading gossip) and active (e.g. arguing, offensive statements) or passive (e.g. ignoring, deliberately not answering phone calls).

The present study results have shown that in the residential care home employee group the incidence of gossip significantly ($p < 0.01$) correlates with workplace bullying (0.28).

In order to reduce conflicts between workers, the following actions are recommended:

- developing clear procedures for reporting and handling of worker complaints,
- management participation in conflict resolution, negotiation and mediation training courses,
- ensuring that workers participate in interpersonal training courses on communication skills and assertive behavior,
- building a psychological contract and introduction of the planned employee rotation system, enabling teamwork (in various personal configurations), based on direct contact and cooperation,
- ensuring that managers at all levels are trained on how to prevent and minimize interpersonal conflicts at work.

5.10.5 ACTIONS TO STRENGTHEN JOB CONTROL AND SOCIAL SUPPORT

The current research has revealed that social support received from management correlates significantly ($p < 0.01$) with development opportunities (Spearman's $\rho = 0.25$), work engagement (0.28), and social climate (0.31), while co-worker social support correlates significantly ($p < 0.01$) with development opportunities (0.28), work engagement (0.25), social climate (0.62), and job satisfaction (0.29), as well as depression (–0.26) and cognitive stress (–0.22). Job control correlates significantly ($p < 0.01$) with development opportunities (0.40), work engagement (0.34), social climate (0.35), and job satisfaction (0.33). For most personnel working with patients/clients, social support reduces the negative impact of stressors at work on mental health and job burnout [Baka 2013]. Therefore, stress prevention programs should aim not only to directly reduce the harmful effects of stressors, but also to strengthen organizational resources (e.g. perceived social support and job control) and individual resources (e.g. positive perception of individual effectiveness, sense of coherence, optimism). Job security and regular social support at all levels enhance worker confidence in effectively coping with problems at work, and promote an optimistic perception of reality. Comprehensive organizational resources (e.g. strong social support) are conducive to the development of individual resources.

The following are examples of potential actions to increase social support at work:

- providing training to management on the role of social support in the workplace and its benefits, e.g. increase in job satisfaction levels and, as a result, increase in employee work engagement and commitment to the organization, and reduced job burnout levels,

- interviewing managers and employees about the role of peer support in coping with stress,
- increasing the availability of "support networks" at work, e.g. greater employee access to senior management,
- organizing self-help groups.

REFERENCES

Ablett, J. R., and R. S. P. Jones. 2007. Resilience and well-being in palliative care staff: A qualitatice study of hospice nurses' experience of work. *Psycho-Oncology* 16(8):733–740. DOI: 10.1002/pon.1130.

Baka, Ł. 2013. Zależności między konfliktami praca-rodzina i rodzina-praca a zdrowiem pielęgniarek. Buforujący efekt wsparcia społecznego. [Relationships between work-family and family-work conflicts and health of nurses: Buffering effects of social support]. *Med Pr* 64(6):775–784. DOI: 10.13075/mp.5893.2013.006.

Baka, Ł. 2017. *Zachowania kontrproduktywne w pracy: Dlaczego pracownicy szkodzą organizacji?* Warszawa: Wydawnictwo Naukowe SCHOLAR.

Cameron, F., and S. Brownie. 2010. Enhancing resilience in registered aged care nurses. *Australas J Ageing* 29(2):66–71. DOI: 10.1111/j.1741-6612.2009.00416.x.

COPSOQ II [Copenhagen Psychosocial Questionnaire II]. 2007. The construction of the scales in COPSOQ II. http://nfa.dk/da/Vaerktoejer/Sporgeskemaer/Copenhagen-Psychosocial-Questionnaire-COPSOQ-II/Engelsk-udgave (accessed November 04, 2019).

Demerouti, E., A. B. Bakker, F. Nachreiner, and W. B. Schaufeli. 2001. The job demands–resources model of burnout. *J Appl Psychol* 86(3):499–512. DOI: 10.1037/0021-9010.86.3.499.

Dz.U. 2008. Nr 237, poz. 1656. 2008. Ustawa z dnia 19 grudnia 2008 r. o emeryturach pomostowych. http://prawo.sejm.gov.pl/isap.nsf/DocDetails.xsp?id=WDU20082371656 (accessed November 04, 2019)

Fengler, J. 2001. *Pomaganie męczy: Wypalenie w pracy zawodowej.* Gdańsk: GWP.

Gallego-Alberto, L., A. Losada, C. Vara, J. Olazarán, R. Muñiz, and K. Pillemer. 2018. Psychosocial predictors of anxiety in nursing home staff. *Clin Gerontol* 41(4):282–292. DOI: 10.1080/07317115.2017.1370056.

Grossman, P., L. Niemann, S. Schmidt, and H. Walach. 2004. Mindfulness-based stress reduction and health benefits: A meta-analysis. *J Psychosomat Res* 57(1):35–43.

Jensen, J. M., P. C. Patel, and J. G. Messersmith. 2013. High-performance work systems and job control. *J Manag* 39(6):1699–1724. DOI: 10.1177/0149206311419663.

Jones, A., C. S. Norman, and B. Wier. 2010. Healthy lifestyle as a coping mechanism for role stress in public accounting. *Behav Res Account* 22(1):21–41. DOI: 10.2308/bria.2010.22.1.21.

Lalak, D., and T. Pilch, eds. 1996. *Elementarne pojęcia pedagogiki i pracy socjalnej.* Warszawa: Wydawnictwo Akademickie "Żak".

Łuczak, A., and D. Żołnierczyk-Zreda. 2002. Praca a stres. *Bezpieczeństwo Pracy – Nauka i Praktyka* 10:2–5.

Malińska, M., A. Namysł, and K. Hildt-Ciupińska. 2012. Promocja zdrowia w miejscu pracy – dobre praktyki. *Bezpieczeństwo Pracy – Nauka i Praktyka* 07:18–21.

Mayo Clinic Staff. 2018. Exercise and stress: Get moving to manage stress. www.mayoclinic.org/healthy-lifestyle/stress-management/in-depth/exercise-and-stress/art-20044469 (accessed November 04, 2019).

McCraty, R., M. Atkinson, and D. Tomasino. 2003. Impact of a workplace stress reduction program on blood pressure and emotional health in hypertensive employees. *J Altern Complement Med* 9(3):355–36. DOI: 10.1089/107555303765551589.

Meisler, G., E. Vigoda-Gadot, and A. Drory. 2017. Stress, psychological strain, and reduced organizational effectiveness: The destructive consequences of the use of intimidation and pressure by supervisors. In *Power, politics, and political skill in job stress (research in occupational stress and well-being*, Vol. 15, eds. C. C. Rosen, and P. L. Perrewé, 51–80. Bingley: Emerald Publishing Limited. DOI: 10.1108/S1479-355520170000015005.

Mockałło, Z., and A. Najmiec. 2017. Stres w pracy z klientem: Źródła, skutki i sposoby przeciwdziałania. *Prewencja i Rehabilitacja* 3–4:1–19. www.zus.pl/documents/1018 2/167752/2017Prewencja_i_rehabilitacja_nr+3_4_2017_49_50/413de773-c8d0-4e9a-9b7b-f8a6e406a4bb (accessed November 04, 2019).

Ogińska-Bulik, N. 2018. Związek między wypaleniem zawodowym i wtórnym stresem traumatycznym wśród pielęgniarek pracujących w opiece paliatywnej. *Psychiatria* 15(2):63–69.

Proper, K. I., B. J. Staal, V. H. Hildebrandt, A. J. van der Beek, and W. van Mechelen. 2002. Effectiveness of physical activity programs at worksites with respect to work-related outcomes. *Scand J Work Environ Health* 28(2):75–84. DOI: 10.5271/sjweh.651.

Rymsza, M. 2012. Pracownicy socjalni i praca socjalna w Polsce. In *Pracownicy socjalni i praca socjalna w Polsce. Między służbą społeczną a urzędem*, ed. M. Rymsza. Warszawa: Instytut Spraw Publicznych.

Schonfeld, I., R. Bianchi, and P. Luehring-Jones. 2017. Consequences of job stress for the mental health of teachers. In *Educator stress: An occupational health perspective*, eds. T. McIntyre, S. McIntyre, and D. Francis, 55–75. Boston: Springer.

Sharma, M., and S. E. Rush. 2014. Mindfulness-based stress reduction as a stress management intervention for healthy individuals: A systematic review. *Evid-Based Complement Altern Med* 19(4):271–286. DOI: 10.1177/2156587214543143.

Spector, P. E., and S. M. Jex. 1998. Development of four self-report measures of job stressors and strain: Interpersonal Conflict at Work Scale, Organizational Constraints Scale, Quantitative Workload Inventory and Physical Symptoms Inventory. *J Occup Health Psychol* 3(4):356–367. DOI: 10.1080/10803548.2015.1116816.

Szmagalski, J. 2009. *Stres i wypalenie zawodowe pracowników socjalnych*. Warszawa: Instytut Rozwoju Służb Społecznych.

Woodhead, E. L., L. Northrop, and B. Edelstein. 2014. Stress, social support, and burnout among long-term care nursing staff. *J Appl Gerontol* 35(1):84–105. DOI: 10.1177/0733464814542465.

Zhang, Y., L. Punnett, B. Mawn, and R. Gore. 2016. Working conditions and mental health of nursing staff in nursing homes. *Issues in Ment Health Nurs* 37(7):485–492. DOI: 10.3109/01612840.2016.1162884.

6 Psychosocial Stressors at Work and Stress Prevention Methods among Medical Staff of Psychiatric and Addiction Treatment Wards

Anna Łuczak

CONTENTS

6.1   INTRODUCTION

According to European Agency for Safety and Health at Work (EU-OSHA), 25% of European workers experience work-related stress all, or most of the working time, and a similar proportion believe that work has a negative impact on their health [EU-OSHA 2014a]. Work-related stress is experienced when the demands of the working environment exceed the worker's ability to cope with those requirements [EU-OSHA 2002]. Occupational stress is closely related to psychosocial risk factors, which include excessive workload and work pace, job insecurity, inflexible shift system, irregular working hours, poor social relations and communication, weak job control, lack of role clarity, poor career development opportunities and *work-family* conflict [Cox 1993].

The effects of work-related stress experiences have various consequences, including in particular, an adverse impact on employee physical and mental health such as depression, cardiovascular diseases, musculoskeletal disorders and diabetes. Attention has been drawn to significant financial costs associated with the treatment of stress-related health outcomes, which in Europe in 2012 amounted to 9% of stress-related and cardiovascular diseases healthcare expenditure, and 1% in 2004 and 2% in 2011 of the European GDP on depression and musculoskeletal disorders expenditure, respectively. Poland, along with Latvia and Estonia, has been at the forefront of healthcare spending on cardiovascular diseases (17%) [EU-OSHA 2014b]. There have also been observed significant business costs resulting from non-health consequences of work-related stress, namely increased absenteeism, staff turnover, and productivity losses.

This chapter presents psychosocial sources of occupational stress among medical staff of psychiatric and addiction treatment wards working in direct contact with patients, in Poland. It also proposes occupational stress prevention methods addressed to this occupational group.

6.2   MEDICAL STAFF IN PSYCHIATRIC HEALTH CARE

In accordance with Article 3 of the Act of 30 August 1991 *on Health Care Institutions* [Dz.U. 2007], medical personnel of psychiatric and addiction treatment wards providing direct patient care in Poland include not only persons performing medical professions, such as doctors and nurses, but also persons entitled to provide health services, i.e. psychologists conducting psychological research, and occupational therapists conducting psychological therapy. In addition, medical staff may include ward nurses and paramedics who participate in the treatment process by performing direct patient care work, including personal care services (patient hygiene procedures, providing assistance to patients in meeting their physiological needs, transporting patients, delivering and serving meals), assisting doctors and nurses in carrying out the examination (e.g. placing and keeping the patient in an appropriate position), and assisting in all activities where the assistance of a third person is required. In special cases, ward nurses and paramedics may use direct coercive measures against the patient (e.g. restraint, compulsory administration of medication or immobilization of the patient).

The specificity of the work performed by medical staff of psychiatric and addiction treatment wards is based on intensive and direct contact with other people (patients, patients' family members, co-workers), resulting from the requirement to provide assistance in various forms: from saving lives, protecting health, and providing constant care for the sick, to cooperation with medical staff members and patients' families. The character of these relations makes the *emotional labor* an integral feature of the profession, whereby emotional regulation is required to display organizationally desired emotions by the employee [Zapf and Holz 2006], or behaviors performed for the benefit of the performer's relationships with others [Pisaniello, Winefield, and Delfabbro 2012] or behaviors improving the emotional well-being of others and creating cooperative and positive social relationships [Strazdins 2000].

Medical personnel of psychiatric healthcare constitute one of the 24 *special character professions* in Poland. These are occupations "requiring particular responsibilities and psychophysical fitness, the ability of which to be properly performed without endangering public safety, including the health or life of others, is reduced before reaching the retirement age as a result of deteriorating psychophysical fitness associated with the ageing process" [Dz.U. 2007]. According to Polish law [*ibid*], performance of special character work duties entitles the employee – while meeting additional conditions, such as age and length of service – to an early retirement.

The World Health Organization has drawn attention to the global changes in the area of psychiatric care, where there has been a shortage of staff and a related problem of a large number of patients per medical staff, and poor working conditions [WHO 2007]. Case studies of doctors who report on their feelings after several years of working with psychiatric patients show that the reason for the experienced professional burnout are excessive job demands, which involve a wide scope of responsibilities, and a lack of support and assistance due to medical staff shortages. This results in fatigue and exhaustion, both physical (including headaches, gastric problems, and sleep disorders) and mental (lack of energy at work, a sense of a lack of purpose in the work, poor job satisfaction, frequent feelings of irritation and difficult interpersonal relations) [Wilczek-Rużyczka 2014]. A report on the mental health care in Poland [Wciórka 2014] provides data on the number of psychiatrists and psychiatric nurses per 100,000 inhabitants, which is lower than the European average, and amounts to 6 doctors and 18.6 nurses, while in the Czech Republic, for example, the respective numbers are 12 doctors and 33 nurses, and in Finland, 22 doctors and 180 nurses.

6.3 PSYCHOSOCIAL STRESSORS AT WORK FOR MEDICAL STAFF OF PSYCHIATRIC WARDS – PRESENT RESEARCH

6.3.1 AIM OF THE STUDY

The aim of the study was to identify sources of stress at work among medical staff of psychiatric and addiction treatment wards providing direct patient care services, based on a current analysis of psychosocial working conditions and quality of life of this professional group in Poland, and to propose appropriate stress-coping support methods.

6.3.2 METHOD

6.3.2.1 Measure

The *Copenhagen Psychosocial Questionnaire II* (COPSOQ II) long version [Pejtersen, Kristensen, and Borg 2010] was used to assess psychosocial working conditions. The questionnaire consists of 41 scales comprising 127 items taking into account the following aspects of work: demands at work (18 items), work organization and job content (17 items), interpersonal relations and leadership (22 items), work-individual interface (17 items), values at workplace level (15 items), health and well-being in the last four weeks (25 items), personality (6 items), and offensive behaviors in the last 12 months (7 items).

Most of the items in COPSOQ II have a five-point response scale: *always, often, sometimes, seldom, never/hardly ever* or *to a very large extent, to a large extent, somewhat, to a small extent, to a very small extent.* All of the COPSOQ II scales are scored 0–100 points. Five-point response scales are scored as follows: 100, 75, 50, 25, 0, while four-point response scales are scored: 100, 66.7, 33.3, 0, respectively.

The psychometric properties of the questionnaire are satisfactory. A study conducted in a group of 3,517 Danish workers has demonstrated the predictive validity of the COPSOQ II – long version [Rugulies, Aust, and Pejtersen 2010]. The reliability studies of the COPSOQ II medium-length version, extended by an additional 25 questions (112 items in total) and conducted among a group of 349 Danish workers using the *interclass correlation* method (ICC), have shown a satisfactory or good reliability (0.70–0.89) except for the *mutual trust between employees* items. Internal consistency, calculated for eight selected scales, has been satisfactory or good (Cronbach's α = 0.75–0.85 for seven scales: *work pace, commitment to the workplace, role clarity, work–family conflict, burnout, stress* and *sleeping troubles*). The test–retest reliability has been satisfactory (0.72–0.81) for six out of eight analyzed scales (*work pace, commitment to the workplace, role clarity, work–family conflict, burnout* and *sleeping troubles*) [Thorsen and Bjorner 2010]. Polish studies [Widerszal-Bazyl 2017], conducted in a group of 7,746 employees (nurses, public servants, teachers and employees of restructured organizations) have shown a satisfactory reliability (Cronbach' α = 0.7–0.91) and validity for eight scales of the questionnaire: *quantitative demands, influence, social support, possibilities for development, meaning of work, quality of leadership, job satisfaction* and *general health perception.*

6.3.2.2 Participants

The study group consisted of 201 persons working as medical staff of psychiatric and addiction treatment wards performing direct patient care work. The majority were women, with n = 160 (79.6%); men were n = 40 (19.9%). One person did not have gender data. The respondent's age was between 26 and 66 years, and the average age was M = 42.2 (SD = 9.21). A large number of persons had completed higher

(72.6%) and secondary education (17.9%). The average length of service in the current occupation was $M = 15.9$ years ($SD = 10.80$). The respondents were employed in the following types of institutions throughout the country: neuropsychiatric hospitals, psychiatric hospitals and hospitals for the nervously ill, psychiatric wards for children and adolescents, daytime psychiatric wards for children and adolescents, addiction treatment wards, daytime alcohol therapy wards, psychiatric health care centers, psychiatric centers, specialist health centers, rehab treatment centers and residential care centers, addiction treatment centers, addiction therapy and alcohol co-dependence counseling centers, and mental health associations. The sample selection was carried out using the quota-sampling method, taking into account the age and gender structure of each institution where the study was conducted.

Most respondents were employed as nurses (27.4%), psychologists, occupational and addiction therapists (10.4% each), physicians (9%) and ward nurses (7%). Moreover, among the respondents there were eight teachers, eight pedagogical employees, six nurses/paramedics, and four social workers. All respondents were employed in the public sector. The vast majority of respondents declared that they performed intellectual work (67.7%). Physical work was performed by 22.4% of respondents, while 6% performed both physical and intellectual work.

The survey was conducted by a social research agency in the period of May–July 2017. Full confidentiality of data and anonymity were preserved. Those respondents who provided an informed consent were asked to fill out the questionnaires and seal them in envelopes, which were subsequently collected by research assistants. All participants were treated in accordance with the Declaration of Helsinki ethical guidelines.

6.4 RESULTS

6.4.1 EMOTIONAL DEMANDS

Due to the absence of COPSOQ questionnaire standardized norms, the study results were analyzed taking as a reference the study of Danish workers ($N = 3,517$), aged 20–59 years, where 52% of respondents were women [COPSOQ II 2007].

The results of the analysis (Table 6.1) has shown that the medical staff of psychiatric wards differs significantly from the Danish study sample in terms of the emotional demands scale [$t(3716) = 14.71$; $p = 0.000$] – the mean emotional demands of the psychiatric care medical staff were significantly higher ($M = 66.45$; $SD = 20.87$) compared to the Danish study group ($M = 40.7$; $SD = 24.3$). The effect size (Cohen's $d = 0.48$) indicates a moderate relationship between the specificity of the study sample (medical psychiatric care staff in Poland/Danish workers) and the level of emotional demands.

Regarding the remaining 21 scales, where there were observed significant differences between the Polish and Danish samples ($p < 0.05$), the Cohen's effect size was low (0.07–0.22). In the light of the above results, significantly higher emotional demands in the Polish sample in comparison with the Danish sample have been considered the primary psychosocial source of stress for the medical staff of psychiatric

TABLE 6.1
The Results of Comparisons of the Polish Sample with Danish Employees Regarding the Scales of the COPSOQ II Questionnaire

	Poland			Denmark			Student's t			
	X	SD	N	X	SD	N	t	df	p	Cohen's d
Demands at work										
Quantitative demands	35.31	17.75	201	40.2	20.5	3517	3.31	3716	0.001	0.11
Work pace	54.77	21.08	201	59.5	19.1	3517	3.40	3716	0.001	0.11
Cognitive demands	64.42	18.77	201	63.9	18.7	3517	0.38	3716	0.701	—
Emotional demands	66.45	20.87	201	40.7	24.3	3517	14.71	3716	0.000	0.48
Demands for hiding emotions	54.33	21.93	201	50.6	20.8	3517	2.46	3716	0.014	0.08
Work organization and job contents										
Influence	45.67	18.76	201	49.8	21.2	3517	2.70	3716	0.007	0.09
Possibilities for development	64.76	20.29	201	65.9	17.6	3517	0.88	3716	0.376	—
Variation	57.09	22.07	201	60.4	21.4	3517	2.13	3716	0.033	0.07
Meaning of work	72.05	17.12	201	73.8	15.8	3517	1.52	3716	0.129	—
Commitment to the workplace	59.9	16.18	201	60.9	20.4	3517	0.68	3716	0.495	—
Interpersonal relations and leadership										
Predictability	58.78	18.41	201	57.7	20.9	3517	0.72	3716	0.473	—
Recognitions (Reward)	60.4	20.54	201	66.2	19.9	3517	4.01	3716	0.000	0.13
Role clarity	75.27	15.89	201	73.5	16.4	3517	1.49	3716	0.136	—
Role conflicts	38.19	19.24	201	42	16.6	3517	3.13	3716	0.002	0.10
Quality of leadership	59.45	23.35	201	55.3	21.1	3517	2.69	3716	0.007	0.09
Social support from colleagues	58.17	20.98	201	57.3	19.7	3517	0.61	3716	0.544	—

(Continued)

TABLE 6.1 (CONTINUED)

The Results of Comparisons of the Polish Sample with Danish Employees Regarding the Scales of the COPSOQ II Questionnaire

	Poland			Denmark			Student's t			Cohen's d
	X	SD	N	X	SD	N	t	df	p	
Social community at work	72.17	18.96	201	78.7	18.9	3517	4.76	3716	0.000	0.16
Social support from supervisor	64.3	24.7	201	61.6	22.4	3517	1.65	3716	0.099	—
Work–individual interface										
Job insecurity	24.42	20.8	201	23.7	20.8	3517	0.48	3716	0.633	—
Job satisfaction	62.42	13.25	201	65.3	18.2	3517	2.21	3716	0.027	0.07
Work–family conflict	35.65	26.15	201	33.5	24.3	3517	1.21	3716	0.225	—
Family–work conflict	10.47	20.74	201	7.6	15.3	3517	2.53	3716	0.011	0.08
Values at workplace level										
Mutual trust between employees	61.08	19.48	201	68.6	16.9	3517	6.08	3716	0.000	0.20
Trust regarding management	63.02	17.05	201	67	17.7	3517	3.11	3716	0.002	0.10
Justice	54.64	16.77	201	59.2	17.7	3517	3.56	3716	0.000	0.12
Social inclusiveness	67.01	15.98	201	67.5	16.3	3517	0.41	3716	0.678	—
Health and well-being										
General health perception	56.59	20.08	201	64.2	23.2	3517	4.55	3716	0.000	0.15
Sleeping troubles	26.9	20.5	201	21.3	19	3517	4.05	3716	0.000	0.13
Burnout	38.77	18.28	201	34.1	18.2	3517	3.54	3716	0.000	0.12
Stress	33.7	17.2	201	26.7	17.7	3517	5.46	3716	0.000	0.18
Depressive symptoms	25.84	15.86	201	21	16.5	3517	4.05	3716	0.000	0.13
Somatic stress symptoms	19.02	15.66	201	17.8	16	3517	1.05	3716	0.293	—
Cognitive stress symptoms	23.32	15.28	201	17.8	17.7	3517	4.33	3716	0.000	0.14
Personality										
Self-efficacy	59.68	17.87	201	67.5	16	3517	6.69	3716	0.000	0.22

wards. Figure 6.1 illustrates the level of different aspects of emotional demands in the medical staff of psychiatric wards study group.

6.4.2 OFFENSIVE BEHAVIORS – THREATS OF VIOLENCE

Parallel to the study of psychosocial sources of stress among medical staff of psychiatric wards, two other occupational groups with emotional job demands, namely personnel of youth rehabilitation centers and youth correctional facilities, G1 (n = 200) and personnel of residential care homes, G2 (n = 200), were also studied in this respect. The intergroup difference significance analysis (the Kruskal–Wallis independent samples test and the Mann–Whitney U test) showed that one of the forms of offensive behaviors, i.e. *threats of violence*, reached the highest level among the medical personnel of psychiatric wards (M_{G3} = 7.91, SD_{G3} = 20.03) group, in comparison to the other two groups (M_{G1} = 2.14, SD_{G1} = 8.25; M_{G2} = 5.78, SD_{G2} = 16.80), (Kruskal–Wallis H test (2, N = 597) = 13.014; p = 0.001). Medical staff of psychiatric wards differed significantly in this regard from the personnel of youth rehabilitation centers and correction facilitates, G1 (U = 17348.500; p = 0.000). The percentage of workers exposed to this type of behavior *once* or *several times* in the preceding year in the medical staff of psychiatric wards group was 14.1% (Figure 6.2) and the perpetrators were mainly patients (16.6% of victims indicated this source – Figure 6.3).

6.4.3 LIFESTYLE – ALCOHOL CONSUMPTION AND PHYSICAL ACTIVITY

A comparison of the medical staff of psychiatric wards with the two above-mentioned occupational groups with emotional job demands revealed another significant

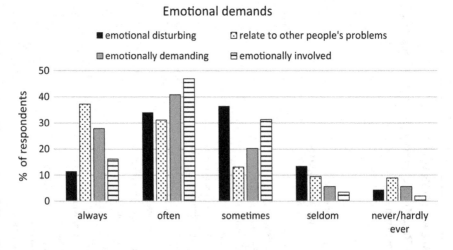

FIGURE 6.1 Emotional demands in the group of medical personnel of psychiatric departments.

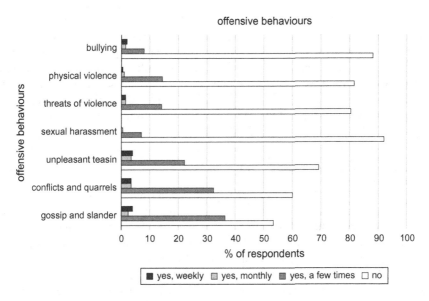

FIGURE 6.2   Exposure to offensive behaviors in the medical staff of psychiatric wards.

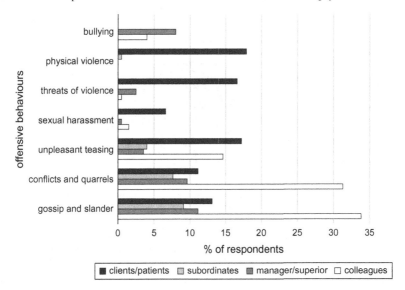

FIGURE 6.3   Source of exposure to offensive behavior and percentage of psychiatric wards exposed in the medical staff group.

difference between the groups in terms of alcohol consumption (Kruskal–Wallis H test (2, N = 592) = 7.36; p = 0.025). The Mann–Whitney U test showed that medical staff of psychiatric wards had significantly more drinks a week (M_{G3} = 0.55, SD_{G3} = 1.42) than the personnel of youth rehabilitation centers and correction facilitates, G1 (M_{G1} = 0.36, SD_{G1} = 1.36), (U = 17745.500; p = 0.029) and the personnel of residential care homes (M_{G2} = 0.23, SD_{G2} = 0.63), (U = 17911.00; p = 0.019).

Figure 6.4 illustrates the problem of physical activity. The results reveal that the largest group of psychiatric care medical staff undertook only light physical activity (e.g. walking, light gardening, light exercises, etc.), one quarter declared intense activity (e.g. fast walking, cycling at high speed or cardio exercises for 2–4 hours a week), whereas the least numerous group opted for an intense physical activity for more than 4 hours a week or for regular, heavy exercises/training sessions. A worrying phenomenon is the fact that 20% of respondents were physically inactive after work, spending leisure time reading newspapers or books or watching television.

6.5 DISCUSSION OF RESULTS

High emotional demands have proved to be the main stressor in the work of medical staff of psychiatric wards. This means that professional duties often place workers in emotionally difficult situations, such as aggressive patient behavior, patient death, suicide attempts or the need to apply direct coercive measures on patients. Emotional demands also arise from the requirement to address other people's personal problems, e.g. conflicts between the patient's family and the patient, or conflicts between patients. These two aspects of emotional demands result in a strong emotional engagement in the performed duties.

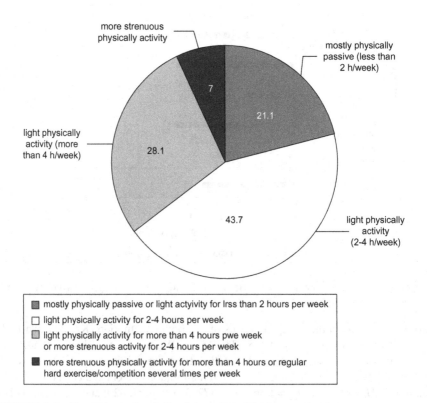

FIGURE 6.4   Physical exercise during leisure time [% of respondents].

The high score in terms of emotional demands observed in the Polish sample is consistent with previous research findings indicating that frequent conflicts with patients, exposure to patient aggression, participation in the disease process, contact with death, and ethical dilemmas, are the main source of stress and its adverse health consequences among medical staff of psychiatric wards [Bakker, Demerouti, and Euwema 2005; Alkrisat and Alatrash 2016; Ando and Kawano 2016]. The emotional burden carried by this professional group has an impact on individual decision-making powers, defined as personal influence or lack thereof in decisions affecting the individual, and therefore on the level of job control, the way the tasks are performed, and on participation in decisions made at the workplace [Tuvesson, Eklund, and Wann-Hansson 2012].

Significantly higher emotional demands in the studied Polish sample in comparison to the general population of Danish employees stem from the specific nature of the special character job, where emotional labor is an inherent part of the work.

The second significant stressor is offensive behaviors, whereby the most troublesome have been identified as threats of violence. Previous research in the field has drawn attention to the phenomenon of increased violence against the medical staff of psychiatric wards, and thus also to the need for research into the development of effective methods to improve safety of the employees [Moylan and Cullinan 2011; Allen 2013; Koukia and Zyga 2013; Itzhaki et al. 2015; Da'seh and Obaid 2017; Zarea et al. 2017].

The main form of violence has been identified as patient aggression. Its experience often forces the staff to devote considerable attention to their own safety and entails social costs such as sick leaves, changing jobs, early retirement and even quitting the profession.

In Poland, patient aggression in psychiatric establishments has also been a significant problem. A study carried out among medical staff of psychiatric hospital wards showed that active aggressive patient behavior was a basic stressor at work, with 90% of respondents being victims of such aggression, 95% witnessing aggression against other workers, and 97% witnessing aggression directed at other patients [Rejek and Szmigiel 2015]. Other studies conducted among psychiatric ward nurses demonstrated that 78% of respondents experienced physical aggression from patients in the form of hand smacks, leg kicks, pushing, hitting with a cup, pinching, and, most often, injuries to upper and lower limbs [Markiewicz 2012]. However, a survey conducted in only one hospital for neurotically and mentally ill patients showed that 27 out of 30 medical personnel who took part in the survey admitted to the experience of patient aggression in the form of cursing, insults, taunts, intimidation, and destruction of hospital equipment, with more than half of respondents having to deal with patient aggression every day [Berent et al. 2009].

The study presented in this chapter has revealed predominant threats of violence. Notably, over 14% of respondents admitted that during the 12 months preceding the survey they had been exposed several times not only to threats of violence but also to acts of physical violence.

When analyzing psychosocial sources of stress in the work of medical staff of psychiatric wards, two lifestyle aspects that distinguish this occupational group should be taken into account, namely alcohol consumption and physical activity. Although almost 80% of employees declared abstinence from alcohol, a significant intra-group variation has been observed (the standard deviation values exceeded the mean value). The results revealed that 8.5% of respondents drank 1 glass of strong alcohol or 1 drink per week, while 5% had from 4 to 10 drinks per week. Regarding physical activity, about 20% of employees declared physical inactivity during their free time. Significantly higher consumption of spirits may be considered a result of stress, while poor physical activity may significantly reduce the ability to cope with stress at work.

6.6   WORK-RELATED STRESS-COPING SUPPORT METHODS

The following stress prevention methods aimed at medical staff of psychiatric wards are primarily employee-oriented and are designed to sensitize the employee to stress symptoms, to learn how to cope with stress, to discover and appreciate individual skill potential, and to use it in the process of self-development and positive transformation of the social environment. The chapter also mentions organization-oriented methods to create a safe working environment conducive to the health of employees.

6.7   EMOTIONAL BURDEN-RELATED STRESS
PREVENTION METHODS

The study presented in the current chapter has shown that the main problem and a potential source of stress in the group of psychiatric care medical staff is high emotional demands. The correlation analysis has proved that although high emotional demands in this occupational group significantly correlate ($p < 0.001$) with such positive aspects of work as personal development opportunities (Spearman's Rho = 0.44), diversity of work tasks (0.36) and importance of work performed (0.38), they are also significantly associated ($p < 0.001$) with adverse psychosocial working conditions such as obtaining contradictory job demands concerning working methods – role conflict (0.33), with a strong work engagement at the expense of family life – work–home conflict (0.43), burnout (0.38), stress (0.33), self-assessed fair and respectful treatment (–0.27) and with conflicts at work (0.22; $p < 0.01$). In light of these results, it seems appropriate to recommend the following methods of stress prevention at work resulting from emotional stress.

6.7.1   MINDFULNESS-BASED STRESS REDUCTION TRAINING

An effective way to reduce stress resulting from emotional work engagement of medical staff of psychiatric wards is *Mindfulness-Based Stress Reduction* (MBSR). Mindfulness means attentiveness, which consists in deliberately or consciously directing one's attention to what is happening and what one feels "here and now". The MBSR training has been designed for persons who experience stress-coping difficulties and negative emotions. Its effectiveness has been confirmed by many studies, including a study conducted in a group of 50 nursing students in Korea [Song and Lindquist 2015]. In this study, the MBSR training took the form of two-hour weekly sessions lasting eight weeks. The results showed that MBSR was an effective, nonpharmacological way to reduce stress, depression and anxiety, also improving attention among the study participants.

A similar result was obtained in other studies conducted in a group of Korean nursing students, where attention training was based on meditation, whereby stress, anxiety, and depression were assessed using appropriate methods: Psychosocial Wellbeing Index – Short Form (PWI-SF), State-Trait Anxiety Inventory (STAI) and Beck Depression Inventory (BDI). Students attended 8 weekly sessions, lasting from 1.5 to 2 hours. Before starting the training, the participants also took part in a 1.5-hour lecture on stress and stress-coping methods. The results proved that the MBSR training was an effective method to reduce stress and anxiety [Kang, Choi, and Ryu 2009].

The impact of MBSR training on stress reduction was also tested during a pilot project carried out over a 7-week period in a group of 14 first year obstetrics and nursing students [Riet et al. 2015]. Effects were evaluated by a partially structured group interview conducted two weeks after the end of the program. The analysis of the interview results showed improved sleep parameters, greater "attention" to oneself and others, better concentration, and clarity of thought. Students learned to recognize symptoms of increased stress and apply appropriate methods of stress reduction.

Similarly, an MBSR training conducted in a group of 20 nurses and 20 midwives was aimed at improving their mental well-being. The training was based on workshops consisting of 20-minute sessions conducted once a day for 8 weeks, and focus-group interviews. During the workshops, participants discussed their own motivation to participate in the workshop activities, pleasant and stressful situations at work, and their influence on their thoughts, emotions, and experienced stress; they also practiced various concentration techniques and learned how to apply the methods in everyday life. The quantitative analysis of the research results showed a significant improvement in mental health parameters, an increase in the sense of personal coherence, and a lower level of stress among the participants. Moreover, the qualitative analysis revealed a very good reception of the training by the participants, the relaxing effect of the session, increased attention from the participants in everyday situations, and a positive influence of attention to emotions and perception of reality. Also, the form of training was acceptable to the participants and easy to carry out. The authors of the study recommended the MBSR training as an element of workplace culture [Foureur et al. 2013].

6.7.2 Strengthening Mental Resilience

Another method of coping with stress at work is the *Promoting Adult Resilience* (PAR) method, defined as promoting inner strength, or the ability to cope with difficult situations and to break out of mental distress. The core components of mental resilience are courage (defined as perseverance in achieving the set goals), determination (not giving in to difficulties), personal ethics and strength (vitality).

The PAR method consists of seven modules:

- understanding of mental resilience,
- building stress awareness and stress-coping strategies,
- demonstrating the problems associated with speaking and thinking badly about oneself,

- fostering an understanding that one can draw strength from overcoming difficulties,
- strengthening positive relations with other people,
- handling conflict situations,
- generating well-being solutions.

The PAR program can be implemented in the workplace, and two full workshop days are sufficient to deliver all the modules.

Studies that applied the PAR program have been conducted in a group of 29 psychiatric nurses in Australia [Foster, Cuzillo, and Furness 2018]. The program was implemented during two-day workshops. Qualitative data on the resilience knowledge, and the usefulness of the program in terms of acquired skills and their practical application, were collected before the first and after the second workshop day, and three months after the end of the program. This data was gathered using a questionnaire method with open questions, partially structured interviews, and focus-group discussions. The data analysis showed that the most emotionally distressing situations were verbal insults or physical aggression on the part of patients or their families, conflicts between employees, and situations beyond the respondent's control. In addition, the study participants became aware of mental resilience as not solely an ability to cope with stress, to control emotions and to overcome the encountered obstacles, but also as an ability to learn, discover and develop personal potential. The participants also had an opportunity to learn from each other during joint discussions, to strengthen their ties with colleagues and, while listening to the problems of others, to realize that they were not alone in experiencing stress at work. The study also revealed that participation in the program enhanced individual resilience through learning about effective tools, realizing that one can learn from stress experiences (post-traumatic growth), emphasizing the importance of taking care of personal well-being and the well-being of co-workers, and that resilience-strengthening methods could be effective in both work and home environments. The respondents also reported they had learned to treat stressors not as an obstacle, but as a challenge of coping with stress and controlling personal emotional response. Other benefits mentioned by the participating nurses included improved job quality, self-esteem, ability to cope with stressful situations, understanding of importance of empathy in interpersonal relations, and resilience to excessive criticism. The research also suggests that the resilience enhancement program benefits not only individuals but also entire teams (positive teamwork culture), the organization (employee well-being culture), and the occupational group (greater professional identity).

Similarly, the results of an Australian survey of nurses and midwives ($N = 14$) have shown that the resilience enhancement program has positive effects both on the individual and on the company as a whole [McDonald et al. 2013]. The program lasted six months and consisted of one-day workshops conducted once a month. During each workshop, two of the following issues related to strengthening resilience were discussed:

- nurturing and maintaining positive social relations,
- mentoring as a partnership relationship between e.g. a supervisor and an employee, aimed at discovering and developing the employee's potential,

- positive thinking,
- so-called "mental hardiness",
- intellectual flexibility,
- emotional intelligence,
- life balance,
- spirituality,
- caution,
- critical thinking.

Data was collected using a partially structured direct interview method in three intervals: before the start of the workshop (awareness of basic problems at work), immediately after the end of the workshop (impact of the training on the individual resilience of the participants), and six months after the end of the resilience enhancement program (long-term effect of the training). The information obtained from the workshop participants enabled the identification of the following individual benefits of the workshop participants:

- the possibility of practical training in conditions conducive to an exchange of experiences and cooperation, and in situations devoid of direct reporting and professional hierarchy,
- the possibility of creative self-expression through art, e.g. painting, drawing, prose, poetry, etc.,
- the experience of new thoughts and behaviors, with the possibility to reflect on one's own life and health the motivation to change existing habits or the life path.

Moreover, professional benefits included an increased assertiveness at work (greater awareness of one's own autonomy and professional self-accomplishment), satisfying social relations at work (greater tendency to reciprocate the support received), greater professionalism (responding with understanding rather than strong emotions in a situation where co-workers have different views on work), understanding the importance of rest breaks and relaxation for the quality of work outcomes, and a sense of both professional accomplishment and satisfaction in other areas of life. According to the authors of the study, the method used to strengthen resilience proved to be effective and helpful in increasing the individual potential of nurses and midwives, and its effects were long-lasting.

Çam and Büyükbayram [2017] reviewed in their study research published between 2007 and 2016 on resilience strengthening strategies and resilience-related factors among nurses. The review showed that high resilience is associated with a professional attitude and has a positive impact on personal life and professional achievements. The authors proposed to create mental resilience development opportunities for nurses as part of undergraduate or postgraduate studies, including such resilience aspects as fostering positive social relations, critical and creative thinking, strengthening self-efficacy, empathy, and ethics, and developing emotional intelligence. Also, environmental factors conducive to a greater resilience have been identified, such as an employee developing personal interests in leisure time (e.g. music, reading, photography, physical activity, yoga, etc.), management support in solving problems (e.g. meetings providing space for signaling and discussing current problems in the workplace, experience sharing among employees, mutual information about publications raising professional knowledge), and celebrating individual successes in the work team, etc.

The resilience enhancement program also proved to be effective for the intervention practices of 27 U.S. emergency nurses from academic hospital emergency departments [Maeler et al. 2014]. The resilience training was based on two-day workshops and lasted twelve weeks. During the workshops, the most stressful situations at work were discussed, and behavioral and cognitive therapy sessions were conducted relating to traumatic events taking place at that time. Equally, attention training, relaxation exercises, and aerobics sessions were introduced. Moreover, the participants maintained a diary of delicate issues, such as situations when they felt uncomfortable, recorded once a week. The study results analysis showed a statistically significant reduction in the levels of depression and post-traumatic stress symptoms as a result of the completed training. The participants also declared that the resilience workshops had been a good opportunity to discuss the most important work-related problems among co-workers, that the therapeutic sessions had helped in coping with traumatic events (e.g. patient's death), and that the physical exercises and other health practices had led to an enhanced understanding of the work–life balance and encouraged them to maintain positive health habits.

6.7.3 EMOTIONAL INTELLIGENCE DEVELOPMENT TRAINING

Another method of reducing occupational stress in professions where the emotional aspect of interpersonal relations constitutes an integral part of the job is a training aimed at developing emotional intelligence, understood as the ability to feel emotions and feelings, and understanding and managing information contained in emotions. A Polish study conducted in a group of 330 persons performing services sector professions such as doctors, nurses, teachers, court superintendents, and managers showed a significant negative correlation between emotional intelligence and stress at work [Oginska-Bulik 2005]. Although this relationship was at a low level ($r = -0.23$; $p < 0.001$), the buffering effect of emotional intelligence in the prevention of negative health effects of stress was observed, particularly in relation to depression symptoms. The same size correlation coefficient between emotional intelligence, especially in terms of self-awareness, self-control, and work-related stress, was obtained in a study conducted among teaching staff at the University of Medical Sciences in Iran [Yamani, Shahabi, and Haghani 2014]. The authors of both studies suggest the need to develop stress-prevention programs at work that include raising the level of emotional intelligence, especially in the case of those jobs and occupations where the element of strong emotions, resulting from interpersonal relations, constitutes the essence of the profession.

6.8 AGGRESSIVE PATIENT BEHAVIOR-RELATED STRESS-PREVENTION METHODS

The current study results presented in this chapter have proved an exposure to negative patient behaviors such as physical violence and threats of violence among the medical staff of psychiatric wards. Intensive and direct contact, as well as the requirement to apply various forms of direct coercion to patients in psychiatric establishments, indicates the need to include methods to counteract the risks in stress management programs. Such a need is particularly justified as the correlation analyses have shown statistically significant relationships ($p < 0.01$) between patient physical violence experienced at work, and the growing work–family conflict observed among the medical personnel of psychiatric wards (Spearman's Rho = 0.22), as well as between patient threats of violence and harassment (0.23), emotional demands (0.21), hiding emotions demands (0.21), and work–family conflict (0.27; $p < 0.001$). Moreover, previous research has drawn attention to the phenomenon of exacerbated violence against the medical staff of psychiatric wards, and thus also to the need for investigating the development of effective methods to improve employee safety. The need for staff-oriented measures has been emphasized, including, in particular, the education of all nurses in the process of exacerbated aggression, the anticipation of violence, and effective intervention measures at various stages of the violence cycle, as in most cases aggression develops according to a predictable pattern. Nurses need to be educated in effective, and at the same time least restrictive, methods of intervention during the initial phase of the aggression process. When patient aggression is sudden or difficult to contain, the nurse must feel confident using coercive measures (e.g. immobilization of the patient, administration of medication) if safety is to be maintained. Training in safe and effective techniques should be available to the staff of acute psychiatric wards. Another example of staff-oriented action is a provision of support to nurses who have been harmed by patient aggression. Examples of measures aimed at organizational changes have also been defined, such as the need for the workplace management to develop a clear and unambiguous security policy in this area [Moylan and Cullinan 2011]. The following actions are therefore recommended.

6.8.1 EDUCATIONAL TRAINING

Da'seh and Obaid [2017], who, based on a literature review, have identified the following risk factors conducive to workplace aggression, point to the need for personnel-oriented action to reduce the risk of exposure to negative patient behaviors:

- patient-related factors:
  - previous episodes of aggression,
  - drugs and alcohol abuse,
  - type of mental illness (schizophrenia, depression, bipolar affective disorders).
- personnel-related factors:
  - a higher level of anxiety among psychiatric ward nurses,
  - a shorter service in psychiatric wards,
  - frustration at work,
  - susceptibility to harsh judgments,
  - hasty and premature reactions,
  - inconsistent attitudes in relations with patients,

- excessive workload hindering an in-depth observation of the patient,
- neglecting frustrated and angry patients,
- confronting patients in the presence of others,
- autocracy,
- lack of training in handling aggressive patient behaviors.
- environmental factors:
  - overcrowded wards,
  - poor building facilities, lighting, and ventilation,
  - inappropriate personnel attitude toward patients,
  - lack of patient entertainment schemes, boredom felt by patients.

The study concludes that prevention of violence in the workplace is essential. Aggression-handling training is a prerequisite, e.g. verbal and non-verbal communication reducing the level of anger among patients, conflict/anger/aggression de-escalation techniques, ensuring respectful treatment of patients and safe conditions, and calm and cautious measures being a signal to the patient that the nurse will not hurt him. The medical staff of psychiatric wards should comprehensively assess the risk of violence, taking into account the patient risk factors, including such aspects as: previous incidents of violence, alcohol and/or drug abuse, male gender and age below 35 years, previously revealed intentions to harm someone, hidden previous aggressive behavior, symptoms of anger or frustration, and fantasies about violence and possible side-effects of medication. Educational training should cover topics such as causes of violence, recognition of alarming signals, raising social skills of staff, violence reporting, de-escalation and prevention procedures, early intervention methods, patient activity programs to reduce boredom, and implementation of effective legal procedures.

6.8.2 Working Environment Settings

The working environment is one of the most important factors directly related to the phenomenon of violence in psychiatric wards. Overcrowding, noise, lack of fresh air and disorder are conducive to aggressive patient behaviors [Da'seh and Obaid 2017]. The following aspects should be noted:

- appropriate physical working conditions, i.e. appropriate lighting, no smoking in wards and availability of smoking zones for smokers, safe spaces for acutely disturbed patients (e.g. safe-room facilities), strong textiles, reinforced glazing, noise isolation, adequate facilities in toilets and bathrooms, entrances and exits under staff control, moderate temperature and good ventilation, privacy in toilets, and separate areas for men and women (bathrooms, toilets, rooms, etc.).
- established procedures
  In the event of violence, the management should draw up an incident report and provide the victim with the necessary advice, support and even time off work to overcome the psychological consequences of the incident. A violence-prevention program should be developed and made available to staff and a team should be appointed to implement its recommendations.

6.9 HEALTH AND WELL-BEING

The analysis of the current study results has revealed a factor that may significantly reduce the ability to cope with stress at work in the psychiatric ward medical staff group, namely its leading position among the analyzed, special character occupational groups in consumption of spirits, and a significant percentage of persons physically inactive during leisure time (21.1%). Moreover, the correlation analysis has showed significant ($p < 0.01$) health associations with job satisfaction (Spearman's Rho = 0.24) and self-efficacy (0.29; $p < 0.001$) on the one hand, and sleeping problems (–0.38), mental tension (–0.28), cognitive stress (–0.28), professional burnout (–0.26), and depression (–0.26) on the other ($p < 0.001$). Therefore, it seems justified to include promotion of a healthy lifestyle in stress-coping support programs in this occupational group.

6.9.1 WORKPLACE HEALTH PROMOTION

Workplace health promotion is, according to the European Network for Workplace Health Promotion (ENWHP), a collective effort of employers, employees, and society to improve the health and well-being of people at work [ENWHP 2009]. The resulting benefits for both enterprise (e.g. reduction of costs related to sick leave and accidents at work, improvement of the company's image, its position in the market, customer satisfaction, lower employee turnover, and improved productivity) and employees (fewer illnesses and accidents, improvement of health and quality of life, and greater job satisfaction) have been emphasized.

Workplace health promotion is an organizational undertaking by enterprise management. It requires an allocation of specific funds for the development of employee infrastructure (e.g. construction of a football pitch or a gym, availability of relaxation rooms, a healthy food buffet), the purchase of sport equipment, financing a medical package and fitness clubs plans, etc. However, it also entails a shift in the understanding of the enterprise mission and its development vision, where, in addition to the provision of specific services (medical treatment, rehabilitation, etc.), the health and well-being of employees need to be fostered. Therefore, workplace health promotion constitutes a stress-coping support method addressed to employees, but also entailing an organizational change.

It has been noted that the effectiveness of health promotion programs is significantly increased when the introduction of a specific program in a company is preceded by an employee "expectations and needs" assessment in this area. This may take the form of a survey, a review of company data (absenteeism, accident rate, health-screening results) or focus group discussions. Such measures can potentially enable the identification of key areas that should be targeted by health-promotion schemes (e.g. obesity, smoking, alcohol problems) [Malińska, Namysl, and Hildt-Ciupińska 2012]. A review of good practices carried out in Poland [*ibid*] has demonstrated that the following methods of workplace health promotion can be considered effective:

- promoting physical activity at the workplace (e.g. setting up an exercise area, sport clubs, encouraging cycling and walking, and partially or totally financing fitness club subscription plans, swimming pool passes, etc.),

- preventive health check-ups (e.g. provision of comprehensive medical care for workers and their families, preventive vaccination, voluntary health check-ups, etc.),
- promoting healthy eating (workshops, seminars, expert advice),
- stress management workshops, organizing excursions and integration events, flexible working hours, etc.,
- addiction quitting programs (e.g. expert workshops on the latest methods of quitting smoking, motivation bonus for non-smokers),
- employee support groups (assisted by management), fostering of a healthy lifestyle by organizing lectures and workshops, (e.g. on relaxation or detox techniques, etc.).

Equally, workplace health promotion should encompass periodic evaluation of the implemented programs' effectiveness and impact by conducting employee surveys, and monitoring the accident rate, employee turnover, number of sick leaves, and performance. Such an analysis results should be communicated to the company's staff, and the management should be obliged to continuously improve the workplace health-promotion methods.

Research conducted by Kelly et al. [2016] has supported the legitimacy of a healthy lifestyle and stress-management workplace measures. The authors examined the diverse sources of stress at work (patient attacks, patient care conflicts and employee conflicts) and how they affected the well-being of psychiatric ward employees: their physical and mental health, and the perception of security at the workplace. The study involved 323 psychiatric hospital staff members employed in major public psychiatric hospitals in California, 69.5% of whom had been physically attacked at work in the 12 months preceding the study. The results revealed that, except for the experiences of physical aggression, daily stressors such as conflicts with patients and between co-workers were found to have a negative impact on the mental well-being and health outcomes among the employees. Individual health habits of the staff (physical activity, diet, amount and type of alcohol and coffee consumption) were also studied. The study proved that health habits had a significant impact on the physical and mental health of workers: those who had negative health habits were characterized by poorer physical and mental well-being. The authors therefore concluded that hospital management should develop a strategy to encourage healthy lifestyles by, for example, offering programs to support individual or group physical activity, encouraging healthy eating (e.g. healthy meal buffets at the workplace), reducing alcohol and coffee consumption, and providing opportunities for specialist consultation and health care.

6.9.2 Prevention of Alcohol Abuse

Workplace health-promotion can also encompass prevention of alcohol problems. It seems that this component should be included in occupational stress-coping programs addressed to medical personnel of psychiatric wards, as this occupational group has been distinguished by the significantly higher consumption of spirits in comparison to the other two groups analyzed. Moreover, prevention is easier and more cost-effective than eliminating or mitigating the consequences of the addiction.

Prevention of alcohol-related problems has been highlighted by the International Labour Organization and the World Health Organization, both of which carry out projects aimed at promoting the idea of "healthy workplace", including the project entitled "Standard model for preventing alcohol and other addictive abuse among employees and their families", initiated in 1993 [Woydyłło-Osiatyńska 1998]. Research carried out in Scandinavia and Western Europe has shown that among the staff of private companies and public sector establishments, non-alcohol or non-drug users make up about 80% of personnel, while those who happen to exceed a healthy dose of alcohol or other mood-changing substances (e.g. sedatives or sleeping pills) make up about 15%, and those "with problems", i.e. alcohol or drug addicts, make up about 5%. The research authors assigned each of the three employee categories a color (green, yellow and red, respectively), and different strategies for each group were proposed. Among the green category group, the belief in the correctly chosen path was reinforced, and those employees were encouraged to participate in a healthy lifestyle training (rather than alcohol-prevention schemes). The yellow category employees, although they did not have a regular alcohol abuse problem, did record instances of poorer work performance or accidents resulting from alcohol consumption. They abused alcohol but were not addicted yet, and should have therefore been encouraged to pay more attention, reduce drinking, and slow down the pace, because they were at risk of falling into addiction. However, there was a likelihood that, under the influence of reliable information, they would change their alcohol consumption habits. In this case, brochures on the health and social impact of alcohol abuse, and access to self-diagnostic questionnaires to calculate alcohol consumption, proved effective. The red category was made up of alcoholics who required medical treatment. In the case of this group, the Employee Assistance Program (EAP), based on assistance provided to employees addicted to alcohol by sober alcoholics (i.e. people who had previously experienced an alcohol problem), proved to be effective. The EAP provides services from Employee Assistance Consultants, whose role is to talk to an employee who has an alcohol addiction problem and refer him/her to an appropriate facility, and then monitor the progress in quitting the addiction. It should be emphasized that the consultant does not provide therapy services. An important element of this system is the direct supervisors who are trained in identifying persons with alcohol problems on the basis of such symptoms as reduced work performance, numerous work breaks, conflicts with co-workers, unjustified absence or delays, inability to work after weekends or vacations, and drinking or having a hangover at work. The role of the supervisor in this case is to confront the employee against whom justified and documented allegations concerning only his/her work with the consultant have been made. The EAP was successfully introduced in several Polish companies in the 1980s.

6.10   SUMMARY AND CONCLUSIONS

The research on psychosocial working conditions has allowed the identification of current sources of work-related stress among medical staff of psychiatric and addiction treatment wards in Poland. The most important stressors have been high emotional demands and patient aggression. However, additional factors such as physical inactivity during leisure time and alcohol abuse can be both consequences of stress, and contribute to a reduced ability to cope with stress at work.

The proposed stress-prevention methods are aimed at developing personal resources, particularly in terms of building and strengthening individual resilience to stress and emotional strain. It is worth recalling that investing in knowledge and health, i.e. the development of employee personal resources, also contributes to the growth of organizational resources, whereby, for example, having competent and engaged workers who are connected with their company and value their co-workers translates directly into a positive social climate, reduced employee turnover and accident risk, and higher employee performance.

The methods presented in this chapter are based on good practice examples that have proved successful for psychiatric healthcare professionals in many countries. It is therefore recommended that they are systematically implemented in order to create safe working conditions and maintain health in the occupational group where exposure to stress is an integral part of the job.

REFERENCES

Alkrisat, M., and M. Alatrash. 2016. Stress and conscience: Concept clarification. *Online J Health Ethics* 12(1):1–13. DOI: 10.18785/ojhe.1201.02.

Allen, D. E. 2013. Staying safe: Re-examining workplace violence in acute psychiatric settings. *J Psychosoc Nurs Ment Health Serv* 51(9):37–41. DOI: 10.3928/02793695-20130612-04.

Ando, M., and M. Kawano. 2016. Association between moral distress and job satisfaction of Japanese psychiatric nurses. *Asian Pac Isl Nurs J* 1(2):55–60. DOI: 10.9741/23736658.1020.

Bakker, A. B., E. Demerouti, and M. C. Euwema. 2005. Job resources buffer the impact of job demands on burnout. *J Occup Health Psychol* 10(2):170–180. DOI: 10.1037/1076-8998.10.2.170.

Berent, D., O. Pierchała, A. Florkowski, and P. Gałecki. 2009. Aggression of patients against the medical staff of the emergency room of the psychiatric hospital. *Psychiatry Psychother* 5(1–2):13–28. www.psychiatriapsychoterapia.pl/?a=articles_showd=963 (accessed November 07, 2019).

COPSOQ II [Copenhagen Psychosocial Questionnaire II]. 2007. The construction of the scales in COPSOQ II. http://nfa.dk/da/Vaerktoejer/Sporgeskemaer/Copenhagen-Psychosocial-Questionnaire-COPSOQ-II/Engelsk-udgave (accessed November 07, 2019).

Cox, T. 1993. Stress research and stress management: Putting theory to work. HSE contract research report no 61/1993:36-49. Sudbury: HSE Books. www.hse.gov.uk/research/crr_pdf/1993/crr93061.pdf (accessed November 07, 2019).

Çam, O., and A. Büyükbayram. 2017. Nurses' resilience and effective factors. *J Psychiatr Nurs* 8(2):118–126. DOI: 10.14744/phd.2017.75436.

Da'seh, A., and O. Obaid. 2017. Workplace violence: Patient's against staff nurse in mental health care setting. *J Nat Sci Res* 7(24):88–95. www.iiste.org/Journals/index.php/JNSR/article/view/40124/41271 (accessed November 07, 2019).

Dz. U. 2007. Nr 14, poz. 89. Obwieszczenie Marszałka Sejmu Rzeczypospolitej Polskiej z dnia 8 stycznia 2007 r. w sprawie ogłoszenia jednolitego tekstu ustawy o zakładach opieki zdrowotnej. http://prawo.sejm.gov.pl/isap.nsf/DocDetails.xsp?id=WDU20070140089 (accessed November 07, 2019).

ENWHP [European Network for Workplace Health Promotion]. 2009. Workplace health promotion. https://oshwiki.eu/wiki/Workplace_Health_Promotion (accessed November 07, 2019).

EU-OSHA [European Agency for Safety and Health at Work]. 2002. Factsheet 22: Work-related stress. http://osha.europa.eu/en/publications/factsheets/22/view. (accessed November 07, 2019).

EU-OSHA [European Agency for Safety and Health at Work]. 2014a. Psychosocial risk in Europe: Prevalence and strategies for prevention. DOI: 10.2806/70971. https://osha.europa.eu/en/publications/psychosocial-risks-europe-prevalence-and-strategies-prevention (accessed November 07, 2019).

EU-OSHA [European Agency for Safety and Health at Work]. 2014b. Calculating the cost of work-related stress and psychosocial risks. DOI: 10.2802/20493 https://pl.scribd.com/document/247812496/Report-Co-branded-EUROFOUND-and-EU-OSHA (accessed November 07, 2019).

Foster, K., C. Cuzillo, and T. Furness. 2018. Strengthening mental health nurses' resilience through a workplace resilience programme: A qualitative inquiry. *J Psychiatr Ment Health Nurs* 25(5–6):338–348. DOI: 10.1111/jpm.12467.

Foureur, M., K. Besley, G. Burton, N. Yu, and J. Crisp. 2013. Enhancing the resilience of nurses and midwives: Pilot of a mindfulness-based program for increased health, sense of coherence and decreased depression, anxiety and stress. *Contemp Nurse* 45(1):114–125. DOI: 10.5172/conu.2013.45.1.114.

Itzhaki, M., A. Peles-Bortz, H. Kostistky, D. Barnov, V. Filshtinsky, and I. Bluvenstein. 2015. Exposure of mental health nurses to violence associated with job satisfaction, life satisfaction, staff resilience and post-traumatic growth. *Int J Ment Health Nurs* 24(5):403–412. DOI: 10.1111/inm.12151.

Kang, Y. S., S. Y. Choi, and E. Ryu. 2009. The effectiveness of a stress-coping program based on mindfulness meditation on the stress, anxiety and depression experienced by nursing students in Korea. *Nurse Educ Today* 29(5):538–543. DOI: 10.1016/j.nedt.2008.12.003.

Kelly, E. L., K. Fenwick, J. S. Brekke, and R. W. Novaco. 2016. Well-being and safety among inpatient psychiatric staff: The impact of conflict, assault and stress reactivity. *Adm Policy Ment Health* 43(5):703–716. DOI: 10.1007/s10488-015-0683-4.

Koukia, E., and S. Zyga. 2013. Critical cases faced by mental health nurses and assistant nurses in psychiatric hospitals in Greece. *Int J Caring Sci* 6(3):465–471. www.researchgate.net/publication/279994109_Critical_Cases_Faced_by_Mental_Health_Nurses_and_Assistant_Nurses_in_Psychiatric_Hospitals_in_Greece (accessed November 07, 2019).

Maeler, M., D. Conrad, J. Evans et al. 2014. Feasibility and acceptability of a resilience training program for intensive care unit nurses. *Am J Crit Care* 23(6):e97–e105. DOI: 10.4037/ajcc2014747.

Malińska, M., A. Namysl, and K. Hildt-Ciupińska. 2012. Promocja zdrowia w miejscu pracy – dobre praktyki (2). [Promoting workplace health – good practices (2)]. *Bezpieczeństwo Pracy – Nauka i Praktyka* 7:18–21. http://yadda.icm.edu.pl/baztech/element/bwmeta1.element.baztech-article-BPC1-0012-0022/c/Malinska.pdf (accessed November 07, 2019).

Markiewicz, R. 2012. Patients' aggressive behaviour towards nursing staff employed in psychiatric wards. *Curr Probl Psychiatry* 13(2):93–97. https://docplayer.pl/5947921-Zachowania-agresywne-pacjentow-wobec-personelu-pielegniarskiego-zatrudnionego-w-oddzialach-psychiatrycznych-renata-markiewicz.html (accessed November 07, 2019).

McDonald, G., D. Jackson, L. Wilkes, and M. H. Vickers. 2013. Personal resilience in nurses and midwives: Effects of a work-based educational intervention. *Contemp Nurse* 45(1):134–143. DOI: 10.5172/conu.2013.45.1.134.

Moylan, L. B., and M. Cullinan. 2011. Frequency of assault and severity of injury of psychiatric nurses in relations to the nurses' decision to restrain. *Int J Ment Health Nurs* 18(6):526–534. DOI: 10.1111/j.1365-2850.2011.01699.x.

Ogińska-Bulik, N. 2005. Emotional intelligence in the workplace: Exploring its effects in occupational stress and health outcomes in human service workers. *Int J Occup Med Environ Health* 18(2):167–175. www.imp.lodz.pl/upload/oficyna/artykuly/pdf/full/Ogi8-02-05.pdf (accessed November 07, 2019).

Pejtersen, J. H., T. S. Kristensen, and V. Borg. 2010. The second version of the Copenhagen Psychosocial Questionnaire. *Scand J Public Health* 38(Suppl 3):8–24. DOI: 10.1177/1403494809354434.

Pisaniello, S. L., H. R. Winefield, and P. F. Delfabbro. 2012. The influence of emotional labour and emotional work on the occupational health and wellbeing of South Australian hospital nurses. *J Vocat Behav* 80(3):579–591. DOI: 10.1016/j.jvb.2012.01.015.

Rejek, E., and M. Szmigiel. 2015. Staff stress related to the specificity of working in a psychiatric ward. *Nurs Prob* 23(4):515–519. DOI: 10.5603/PP.2015.0084.

Riet, P., R. Rossiter, D. Kirby, T. Dłużewska, and C. Harmon. 2015. Piloting a stress-management and mindfulness program for undergraduate nursing students: Student feedback and lessons learned. *Nurse Educ Today* 35(1):44–49. DOI: 10.1016/j.nedt.2014.05.003.

Rugulies, R., B. Aust, and J. H. Pejtersen. 2010. Do psychosocial work environment factors measured with scales from the Copenhagen Psychosocial Questionnaire predict register-based sickness absence of 3 weeks or more in Denmark? *Scand J Public Health* 38(Suppl. 3):42–50. DOI: 10.1177/1403494809346873.

Song, Y., and R. Lindquist. 2015. Effect of mindfulness-based stress reduction on depression, anxiety and mindfulness in Korean nursing students. *Nurse Educ Today* 35(1):86–90. DOI: 10.1016/j.nedt.2014.06.010.

Strazdins, L. M. 2000. Integrating emotions: Multiple role measurement of emotional work. *Aust J Psychol* 52(1):41–50. DOI: 10.1080/00049530008255366.

Thorsen, S. V., and J. B. Bjorner. 2010. Reliability of the Copenhagen Psychosocial Questionnaire. *Scand J Public Health* 38(Suppl. 3):25–32. DOI: 10.1177/1403494809349859.

Tuvesson, H., M. Eklund, and C. Wann-Hansson. 2012. Stress of conscience among psychiatric nursing staff in relation to environmental and individual factors. *Nurs Ethics* 19(2):208–219. DOI: 10.1177/0969733011419239.

Wciórka, J., ed. 2014. Mental health care in Poland: Challenges, plans, barriers, good practices. RPO report. Warsaw: Office of the Ombudsman. www.rpo.gov.pl/sites/default/files/Ochrona_zdrowia_psychicznego.pdf (accessed November 07, 2019).

WHO [World Health Organization]. 2007. Atlas: Nurses in mental health 2007. Geneva: World Health Organization. https://apps.who.int/iris/bitstream/handle/10665/43701/9789241563451_eng.pdf;jsessionid=B3599FCAD9C2E9BE24DF007533934B0B?sequence=1 (accessed November 07, 2019).

Widerszal-Bazyl, M. 2017. Copenhagen Psychosocial Questionnaire (COPSOQ) – Psychometric properties of selected scales in the Polish version. *Med Pr* 68(3):329–348. DOI: 10.13075/mp.5893.00443.

Wilczek-Rużyczka, E. 2014. *Professional Burnout of Medical Workers*. Warsaw: Wolters Kluwer SA.

Woydyłło-Osiatyńska, E. 1998. Drinking alcohol as a workplace problem. In *WHP: Selected Programs*, ed. A. Gniazdowski, 45–74. Łódź: Institute of Occupational Medicine, Prof. Dr Med. Janusz Nofer, National Centre for WHP.

Yamani, N., M. Shahabi, and F. Haghani. 2014. The relationship between emotional intelligence and job stress in the faculty of medicine in Isfahan University of Medical Sciences. *J Adv Med Educ Prof* 2(1):20–26. www.ncbi.nlm.nih.gov/pmc/articles/PMC4235538/pdf/jamp-2-20.pdf (accessed November 07, 2019).

Zapf, D., and M. Holz. 2006. On the positive and negative effects of emotion work in organization. *Eur J Work Organ Psychol* 15(1):1–28. DOI: 10.1080/13594320500412199.

Zarea, K., M. Fereidooni-Moghadam, S. Baraz, and N. Tahery. 2017. Challenges encountered by nurses working in acute psychiatric wards: A qualitative study in Iran. *Issues Ment Health Nurs* 39(3):244–250. DOI: 10.1080/01612840.2017.1377327.

Index

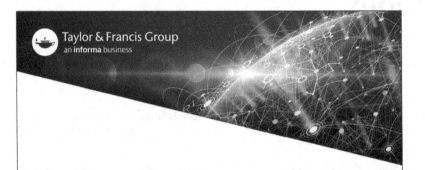

Printed in the United States
by Baker & Taylor Publisher Services